Vaginal birth after caesarean

THE VBAC HANDBOOK

T0131323

Vaginal birth after caesarean

THE VBAC HANDBOOK

Helen Churchill and Wendy Savage

pinter
&
martin

Vaginal Birth After Caesarean
The VBAC Handbook

First published in 2008 by Middlesex University Press
This reprint edition published by Pinter & Martin Ltd 2010
reprinted 2012

Copyright © Helen Churchill

ISBN 978-1-905177-24-0

Also available as ebook.

A CIP catalogue record for this book is available from
The British Library

Interior design by Helen Taylor

Pinter & Martin Limited
Unit 803 Roach Road
4 Roach Road
London EE 2PH

www.pinterandmartin.com

Contents

Introduction

Once a caesarean, always a caesarean?

This statement was made by an American obstetrician in 1916 as a plea for obstetricians to be cautious about using surgical delivery. Unfortunately, in the United States it was taken as an instruction, and so all women had a planned caesarean section for their next baby. This policy wasn't changed until 1978 when public health doctors in the US, alarmed by the tripling of the caesarean section rate in 15 years from five to 16 per cent, called a consensus conference[1] to which 'lay' women were invited. Obstetricians were encouraged to give women the chance to give birth vaginally after one caesarean, and so the phrase VBAC was born. In 1990, as few obstetricians had acted on this and the caesarean section rate was still rising, a target rate of 35 per cent for VBAC was set.[2] It was hoped that the first-time caesarean rate of 24 per cent could be reduced to 15 per cent. Sadly this was not achieved and the US caesarean rate, after a slight reduction, started to climb again at the end of the 1990s.

In the UK, however, obstetricians have always considered it possible for women to aim for vaginal birth after caesarean. In our survey of obstetricians in 1989 only six out of 316 obstetricians followed the US policy of 'once a caesarean, always a caesarean'. Three of these were in Scotland.[3] When we surveyed them again in 2005 we did not ask this question but how they would respond to a woman who had had two caesareans and wanted a VBAC. A third of the 150 obstetricians surveyed said they would be prepared to do this, a third would advise a planned section and the rest were prepared to support the woman with various degrees of enthusiasm. However, one of those commented that he had never had such a request. This confirms the anecdotal evidence that it is commonly believed that once you have had one caesarean, you will require a caesarean for any subsequent babies, known as 'repeat caesareans'. As the number of women having caesareans for their first babies rises, it means that there is an inevitable increase in the number of repeat caesareans. However, there is a wealth of evidence showing that vaginal birth after caesarean is safe for the majority of women and that repeat caesareans may offer no advantage for you or your baby. In 2007 the Royal College of Obstetricians and Gynaecologists published their guideline on 'Vaginal Birth after Previous Caesarean Birth' confirming this view and agreeing that VBAC after two caesareans was reasonable for some women.[4]

The practice of repeat caesareans began in the early 1900s when the rationale behind it had a logical medical basis. At that time the vertical cut in the body of the uterus (classical) predominated and such scars were prone to rupture, particularly during the rigours of labour, because the upper part of the uterus is very muscular. The lower-segment transverse uterine incision underlying the transverse abdominal incision (the Pfannenstiel's or 'bikini-line' cut) in general use today is much less vulnerable to rupture and is associated with lower incidence of maternal and fetal health risks and complications and death. Indeed discussions of uterine rupture are misleading as it is rare. What usually happens is that the scar gives way ('dehiscence' is the medical term) or comes 'unzipped'. There is only a little bleeding and it does not usually result in any serious problems for mother or baby if recognised early and swift action taken to deliver the baby. (See below under 'Risks of VBAC' for a discussion of what happens when the scar opens slightly, p.15).

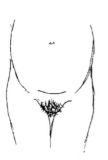

Bikini-line cut

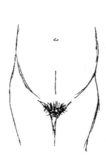

Vertical cut

In the UK in 2000, for the National Caesarean Section Audit,[5] a sample of women were asked questions about their preferences for birth. Overall only 5.3 per cent of women preferred to have a caesarean compared with 8.7 per cent who were told they needed a caesarean for medical reasons; 6.5 per cent had no preference. For women having their first baby, 6.7 per cent were told they needed a caesarean which seems high to us as many of the reasons for needing a caesarean do not occur until labour begins. If one looks at those who had had a previous caesarean, 45 per cent wanted a vaginal delivery, 27.1 per cent were told there were medical reasons for a caesarean and 2.9 per cent had no preference. One small British study reported that many repeat caesareans were performed because women were asking for them, 54 out of 59 women whom the doctors thought were suitable chose a planned caesarean.[6] We have written this handbook because we believe that the key to the increased use of VBAC in the future lies with women being adequately informed about the safety of VBAC combined with accurate unbiased information given by obstetricians and midwives.

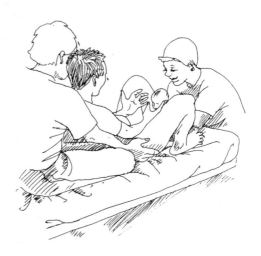

In this book we have set out the case for VBAC offering information and advice on both the benefits and the potential risks. We begin with an overview of the available data on how common VBAC is in 'Rates of VBAC' (p.11). We then provide as much evidence as we could find on the 'Success of VBAC' (p.12) followed by an outline of the potential risks associated with VBAC (p.15) and an examination of cases where VBAC may be considered to be inadvisable (p.19). We balance this discussion with a section on the 'Risks from repeat caesareans' (p.16). You can find information on VBAC after two or more caesareans on page 23 and a discussion of VBAC at home on page 24. The final information section covers what you need to know when making your decision about whether VBAC is the right option for you (p.34). The latter part of the book contains seven VBAC birth stories. Each story begins with a brief overview so you can choose which ones to read if you do not want to read them all. Some of the experiences included here are very positive, others somewhat more traumatic. The common thread is that all the women who have given their stories for this book successfully achieved VBAC and, whilst some of them may have changed some of their decisions, none would have changed their choice to go for VBAC.

A note on the language of labour

When discussing VBAC with health care professionals you may hear terms like 'trial of labour' or 'trial of scar' which refer to them 'allowing' you to 'attempt' vaginal birth. We think that it is unhelpful to women if terms such as 'allowing' a 'trial' are used because of the inference of impending failure. Obstetricians tend to believe that no pregnancy is normal except in retrospect so view the scar with caution, hence using the term 'trial'. To the woman it often seems that she will be allowed to attempt a trial of labour or scar but is not expected to succeed. Couching VBAC in these terms also confers power to the professional to give permission to you to make a decision about how you want to give birth. Such connotations can be disempowering and off-putting so we have tried not to use this type of language in this book. You have a right to decide how you want to give birth and hopefully, armed with information from this book and encouraged by the VBAC birth stories, you will be able to overcome any negative suggestions of needing permission to give birth in a way that you want, if you encounter them. Legally you have the right to decide how to give birth.

Any competent woman who has the capacity to decide may, for religious reasons, other reasons, for rational or irrational reasons or for no reason at all, choose not to have medical intervention, even though the consequence may be the death or serious handicap of the child she bears, or her own death. In that event, the courts do not have the jurisdiction to declare medical intervention lawful and the question of her own best interests objectively considered, does not arise.[7]

VBAC statistics

Rates of VBAC

The old dictum of 'once a caesarean, always a caesarean' appears to be changing. In a survey of obstetricians' views on caesareans that we conducted in 2005, very few said that they agreed with this tradition.[8] Over twenty years ago the World Health Organisation (WHO) stated that 'there is no evidence that caesarean section is required after a previous transverse low segment caesarean section birth.'[9]

In 2000, the VBAC rate for England and Wales was 33 per cent. This is an average and conceals differences in VBAC rates between different regions, from 27 to 38 per cent, and rates ranging from 6 to 64 per cent between individual units. Whether or not you are offered the choice of VBAC will also depend on where you live and which unit you go to. In 2000, 44 per cent of

Table 1 Caesarean section and VBAC rates by region (2000)

Region	CSR %	VBAC %
England	21.5	32.6*
North East	19.3	38.2
North West	19.6	33.7
East Midlands	20.4	34.3
West Midlands	21.8	33.7
Eastern	21.4	32.0
London	24.2	29.6
South East	22.6	31.1
South West	19.4	34.0
Wales	23.8	26.9
Northern Ireland	23.9	23.8
Channel Islands & Isle of Man	24.8	21.8

Source: Thomas & Paranjothy, 2001
* England and Wales

women who had a repeat caesarean said they had been offered a 'trial of labour' and this ranged from 39 to 49 per cent between regions and 8 to 90 per cent between units. The North East region had the highest VBAC rate in Britain, whereas Wales had one of the lowest VBAC rates in Britain.[10]

Success of VBAC

Evidence on the success of VBAC in the UK is scant and most information comes from a few studies in the United States where practice is very different from the United Kingdom. From these it appears that around three-quarters of women with previous caesareans who plan a vaginal birth are successful and it has been concluded that VBAC is safe for the majority of women. Overall VBAC appears to be safer for you and your baby than a planned caesarean and VBAC mothers tend to have the same history and frequency of side effects as mothers with previous vaginal births.[11]

The health risks associated with successful vaginal birth are about one-fifth those of a planned caesarean.[12,13] However, women who have a caesarean after attempting a VBAC will have a slightly higher rate of complications than those who have a planned caesarean, although labour may be good for the baby. Women who achieve successful VBAC have been found in most studies to have fewer health problems after birth than those who go on to have a repeat caesarean including:

- Fewer blood transfusions
- Reduced infection rates
- Shorter hospital stays.[14]

The success of VBAC is related to:
- *The reason for your previous caesarean*
The success of VBAC will be affected by the reason(s) for your previous caesarean. A non-recurrent cause such as breech or fetal distress will have a much higher VBAC success rate than conditions that might recur such as a mismatch between the size of your pelvis and the size of the baby (known medically as cephalopelvic disproportion or CPD). However, two-thirds of women with a history of this can achieve successful VBAC.[15,16,17,18]

- *Later arrival at hospital*
For hospital births, arriving at hospital later in labour usually means that you

are more relaxed and less likely to be subjected to intervention in the progress of your labour. Less intervention in labour means more likelihood of successful vaginal birth. You may find that using a TENS (transcutaneous electrical nerve stimulation) machine or warm bath for pain relief at home will enable you to delay going to hospital.

• *Not having continuous electronic fetal monitoring (EFM)*
This is because EFM restricts your mobility as you are strapped to a machine and often required to lie on a bed. If you cannot move around as you please your labour may not progress or you may experience more discomfort which can affect your perception of the progress of your labour. EFM is sometimes poorly understood or the results can be misread and for this reason it is associated with higher rates of caesarean section. If your attendants want to check your baby with EFM ask them to take their readings and then remove the straps that attach you to the machine so that you can move. Continuous monitoring is recommended by the Royal College of Obstetricians and Gynaecologists but is not mandatory and is not recommended by their US counterparts in the American College of Obstetricians and Gynecologists. Limited research shows that intermittent monitoring every five minutes is just as effective.[19]

• *Epidural anaesthesia at a later stage*
An epidural is a form of regional anaesthesia used to numb the abdomen for routine pain relief during labour and total pain relief during a caesarean. The procedure is done by an anaesthetist who inserts a fine plastic tube between two bones in the lower spine in order to introduce anaesthetic into the spine. Fetal monitoring (EFM) is usually used if there is an epidural because your blood pressure may fall and this can affect your baby and, as stated above, the use of fetal monitoring also affects your chances of successful vaginal birth. If an epidural is to be used it appears that VBAC is more likely to be successful if the epidural is administered at a later stage in labour, i.e. after the cervix has dilated to at least 4cm.

• *Not being induced or having your labour accelerated*
Induction speeds up labour and some researchers think it increases the risk of the scar coming apart.[20] (See discussion of induction on page 21.) Acceleration of labour by artificial rupture of the membranes (ARM) will also speed up labour and may adversely affect VBAC success.

• *Previous vaginal births*
If you have previously given birth vaginally then you are more likely to succeed at VBAC. Your chances of successful VBAC with your current pregnancy are increased if your previous vaginal birth was after your caesarean.[21,22,23,24]

• *Being able to eat and drink in labour*
There appears to be no benefit in restricting food and drink intake during labour as appears to be the 'policy' in some hospitals. There is no harmful effect of eating and drinking in labour and it can help to keep up your energy levels so long as you are sensible about what you eat. Remember that meats and high-fat foods can be heavy on your digestive system so choose carbohydrates that will give a long, slow release of energy. Drink plenty of fluids so that you do not become dehydrated.

• *Being able to move around in labour*
Women report that when you are able move around as you please during labour it helps your labour to progress and you may be able to find more comfortable positions in which to work with your contractions. Try to listen to what your body tells you to do – and do it!

• *No time limits on labour*
It is better for you if you can labour at your own pace and do not feel pressured by time restrictions. Strict adherence to time limits in labour adversely affects its progress because it puts pressure on you. You may begin to feel disempowered or, if you are told that you are taking too long, you may begin to worry that something is not right. Women are more likely to labour successfully, including VBAC, when no time limits are placed on labour.

• *Continuity of care*
Being able to labour attended by health care professionals that you know and with whom you have been able to build a relationship increases your chances of successful VBAC. Staff changes on the labour ward appear to disconcert labouring women and have an adverse effect on the progress of labour.

• *Care from midwives*
When women labour with midwives they have fewer interventions including caesarean section, thus the key to successful VBAC is to leave your care in the hands of midwives for as long as possible.[25,26]

Comparative risks of VBAC and caesarean

Risks of VBAC

Much of the discussion on the relative benefits and disadvantages of planning a vaginal birth after a previous caesarean centres on the perceived risk of the uterus rupturing during labour because it is scarred. As mentioned above, uterine rupture is extremely rare – what is more likely to happen is that the scar may come apart slightly. But it must be remembered that there are many more complications of pregnancy and labour that are far more likely to occur than the uterus rupturing or the scar opening. What is more, there is now a wealth of evidence to support the safety of VBAC.

• *When the scar comes apart*

The UK's National Institute for Clinical Excellence (NICE) guidelines put the risk of the scar opening during labour at 3.5 per 1,000 for women going for a VBAC compared with 1.2 per 1,000 women having a planned caesarean.[27] In the United States, the National Institute of Child Health and Human Development (NICHD) study found higher rates than this but it has been suggested that some enthusiasts in the US were pushing women to the limit and thus had higher rates of scar dehiscence and rupture.[28] The NICE data suggest that only two women in every 1,000 are more likely to experience the scar opening if they choose VBAC than if they opt for a repeat caesarean. However, another authoritative study reported that the possibility of the scar coming apart or rupturing was likely to occur in fewer than 2 per cent of planned VBACs and that this rate was the same for planned repeat caesareans. Where the scar does come apart it is usually slight and does not represent a health risk. Serious wound opening is a rare complication of labour after a previous caesarean[29] and we believe that the benefits of VBAC for you and your baby outweigh this small risk.

It has been suggested that the risk of rupture could be predicted by sonographic assessment of the lower uterine segment thickness.[30] In France and Canada a minority of obstetricians measure the thickness of the uterine scar with ultrasound before agreeing to a VBAC but no randomised controlled trial has been done and one study showed no difference in either the rate of scar dehiscence or proportion of women giving birth normally. In another study the scar could be seen in only a quarter of women and this is not routine practice in the UK. However, if you have an obstetrician who does not agree with your wish to have a VBAC you might try this approach to convince her/him it is safe – although it might be better to find another obstetrician!

- *If the VBAC is not successful*
An unsuccessful labour which ends in caesarean section can carry twice the health problems of a planned repeat caesarean[31] and some complications such as bladder and bowel injury (through laceration) may be higher amongst women who have a caesarean after a planned VBAC.[32] However, the 70–80 per cent of planned VBACs that are successful carry lower rates of health problems meaning that it is better for you to plan a VBAC than a repeat caesarean.[33]

Risks from repeat caesareans

Routine repeat caesarean section is associated with higher risks of complications and more potential problems than VBAC[34] and offers no advantage to you or your baby.

Some of the complications associated with repeat caesareans are:

- Bladder injury at time of repeat caesarean.[35,36]
- Increased risk of bleeding (haemorrhage).
- Blood transfusions and fever after the birth are more common in women who have repeat caesareans.[37]
- Increased risk of emergency hysterectomy. One study put the risk of emergency hysterectomy at one in 90 for women with one previous caesarean having a repeat operation.[38]
- Some women may become shocked after surgery, usually because of blood loss.
- Thromboembolism. This is where clots in the veins cause blockage (or partial blockage) in the blood stream following surgery.

- Higher health risks for the baby.[39] Two recent US papers suggest that more babies died after caesareans done without a medical reason.[40, 41]
- Repeat caesareans may increase risk of maternal death.[42] Caesareans have always been associated with slightly higher maternal death rates although the extent to which this is due to the condition for which the caesarean was performed or to the operation itself is unclear. In the UK between 2000 and 2002 the fatality rate for vaginal birth was 0.004 per cent, considerably less than for caesarean section at 0.17 per cent.[43]

The incidence of some conditions increases with the number of caesareans you have and, as such, repeat caesareans can increase the chances of future problems such as:

- **Placenta praevia:** this means that the placenta is in the wrong position, usually in the lower part of the uterus rather than the upper. If the placenta completely covers the cervix or encroaches on it, bleeding during labour could be fatal and another caesarean will be necessary. The risk of placenta praevia and abruption (see below) are both increased after a first caesarean and the risk of praevia increases with every caesarean you have.[44]

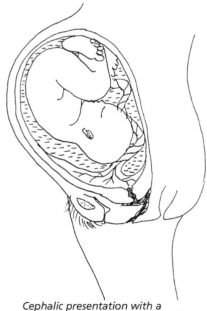

- **Placenta accreta:** this is where the placenta burrows into the uterine wall. The rate of placenta accreta is higher for women with previous caesareans. It is usually found in combination with placenta praevia and usually only checked for if placenta praevia is diagnosed. It has been suggested that the risk of placenta accreta is increased if the placenta implants over the scar from the previous caesarean.[45] The location of implantation can

Cephalic presentation with a grade 3–4 placenta praevia

be determined by scan and if it is clear of the scar you can rule this out as a risk.

• **Placenta abruption:** that is, the premature separation of the placenta from the uterus. Like placenta praevia, the risk of abruption is increased after a first caesarean[46] but it is not clear why this happens.

• **Ectopic pregnancy:** a pregnancy that embeds somewhere other than the uterus, often in the fallopian tubes. This is because there is a higher risk of infection and adhesion (where parts of tissue stick together) following surgery and these may affect the fallopian tubes and so increase the risk of ectopic pregnancy.

There are risks associated with caesarean section and these rise with the number of caesareans you have. What this means is that decisions regarding VBAC versus repeat caesareans need to include consideration of your future plans in terms of whether you intend to have more children. If you plan to have more children, you should seriously consider VBAC as it has been suggested that each caesarean shifts some of the risks from your current pregnancy on to your future births.[47]

Is VBAC ever inadvisable?

There are very few situations or conditions for which VBAC would be completely inadvisable ('contraindications' is the medical term). Again the reason for your previous caesarean(s) will be an important pointer here. Pre-existing conditions or those likely to recur may mean that VBAC is inadvisable but non-recurring conditions will not. VBAC rates are lowest when the previous caesarean section was for cephalopelvic disproportion or lack of progress (failure to progress).[48] Whilst having a long labour is not necessarily a recurring condition, there may be a small number of women who do not labour well particularly if they are sensitive to the noisy, busy, harshly lit labour ward. Even so, successful vaginal birth was achieved in more than 50 per cent of women in published studies and in over 75 per cent of women in one large study where previous caesarean section had been for one of these indications.[49,50]

- *Number of prior caesareans*

One study has suggested that the rate of successful VBAC decreases with increasing numbers of prior caesareans.[51] But this should not put you off planning a VBAC if you think it is the right decision for you. The anecdotal evidence in the birth stories in this book demonstrates that VBAC is possible after two, and even four, prior caesareans.

- *Twins*

It seems that women carrying twins are less likely to plan a VBAC although there is no evidence to suggest that they are more likely to fail a VBAC[52,53] or have increased rates of illness or complications for mother or child.[54] One study reported a success rate of nearly 80 per cent for women carrying twins who planned a VBAC.[55] However, as with women who do not have previous caesareans, the position of the babies in the womb and their weight may have an impact on VBAC success. For example it has been suggested that twins in the vertex/vertex position (both head down) with predicted weights greater than or equal to 2,000g (just over 70oz or four pounds) are the best candidates for vaginal birth of both twins.[56] Obstetricians vary in their approach to non-vertex twin pairs in women who do not have a scarred uterus so their approach to women planning VBAC will be equally variable. If your obstetrician is not happy with you planning a VBAC for non-vertex twins, you could ask for a second opinion or change obstetricians.

- *Pre-eclampsia (PET) and gestational hypertension (GH)*
Pre-eclampsia is a condition arising during pregnancy the symptoms of which are increased blood pressure often accompanied by swelling of the limbs and protein in the urine. The only 'cure' is birth of the baby. If the condition is severe this is usually done by caesarean. If left untreated, PET could cause fits in the mother and cut off the oxygen supply to the baby. Gestational hypertension means that your blood pressure is abnormally high as a result of your pregnancy. Women with PET or GH do not appear to suffer higher risks when going for VBAC but because of the perceived problems, women with GH are less likely to plan VBAC. PET has been associated with a higher VBAC failure rate but overall the VBAC success rate is still relatively high in women with PET.[57]

- *Maternal age*
One study showed that maternal age may affect the success of VBAC. Women older than 35 who had not previously given birth vaginally were found to be more likely not to succeed at VBAC.[58] How much of this lack of success is biological or physiological and how much obstetricians' distress or influence we do not know.

- *Obesity*
One study reported that women who weighed under 14 stone had a VBAC success rate of almost 82 per cent, for those between 14 and 21 stone it was 57 per cent. However, the success rate for women over 21 stone was only 13 per cent.[59] To what extent we can use this data as a guide is unclear as the researchers for this study did not take into account the higher number of previous vaginal births in the women weighing under 14 stone and we know that this increases the success of VBAC. Thus the extent to which weight or body mass index (BMI) affects VBAC success is unclear. Whilst it has been suggested that maternal obesity (being defined as having a BMI over 30) may adversely affect VBAC success[60,61] and more obese women fail at VBAC,[62] there appears to be no physiological explanation for this.[63]

• *Induction*
Some studies have suggested that induction of labour is associated with higher rates of VBAC failure[64] and may lead to the uterus rupturing or the scar coming apart[65,66] more than in spontaneous labour, and this may lead to caesarean section.[67] It appears that the 'type' of induction may have a bearing here. Induction of labour using prostaglandins or misoprostol may increase the risk of uterine rupture in women with previous caesarean births[68] and dinoprostone (used to prepare the cervix for induction) has been associated with a small (but not significant) increase in uterine rupture.[69] However, induction using a transcervical Foley catheter may not increase the risk.[70] Acceleration of labour using an oxytocin drip may mean that some babies become distressed as a result of their oxygen supply being reduced by the stronger contractions that accompany induction which may mean that a repeat caesarean is recommended. It appears that more women achieve successful VBAC after induction when their babies are in the 'normal' position for birth (occipito-anterior position) and when they have had more than one previous birth.[71] We would suggest that you should try to avoid induction if possible.

• *Large baby*
Having a large baby should not affect your success with VBAC and does not necessarily mean that VBAC is inadvisable.[72,73] The size of your baby in relation to your pelvis is important but few women raised in Britain have small pelvises these days in contrast to the Victorian period when poor nutrition, principally rickets, meant that women had very small pelvises. One study showed that women with large babies can safely achieve VBAC[74] although another study suggested that the risk of failure may be increased.[75]

• *Diabetes*
Gestational diabetes is a condition whereby a woman's body does not produce enough insulin during pregnancy. Modern maternity care has made all forms of diabetes less hazardous for both mothers and babies. If you have been diagnosed with diabetes as a condition of your pregnancy and you are controlling it with diet, you should be able to achieve VBAC.[76]

The key is to make sure you have as much information about your condition as you can. Find health care professionals who are supportive of your choices and decisions who will discuss your options and the best course of action.

There are few situations or conditions that prevent successful VBAC and it should be successful in the majority of cases.

Other types of VBAC

Vaginal birth after two or more caesareans

Vaginal birth after two caesareans is usually abbreviated to VBA2C, after three to VBA3C and so on. The information on planned labours after two or more previous caesarean sections is sparse and can be contradictory. Some researchers suggest that the rate of successful VBAC is no worse, and the risks no higher, for women with two or more prior caesareans than those with only one. Other studies have concluded that planned VBACs are less successful and risks greater.[77] There is some evidence to suggest that rates of successful VBAC decrease with increasing numbers of prior caesareans,[78] although you should not be discouraged from planning VBAC if you have two or more previous caesareans. Many women have achieved successful vaginal births after two or more caesareans (see the birth stories in this book, pages 51–82).

A survey we carried out in 2005 of 150 consultant obstetricians showed that over a third said they would advise another caesarean after two previous caesareans. One consultant stated that he had never had such a request, another said that he would tell the women to 'be sensible' and a third said that in such a case the woman should 'find another obstetrician'. Another said 'The consensus is No but it is not written in stone'. Those opposing a vaginal birth often mentioned the possibility of rupture of the previous scar, although they had different figures for the likely risk. One said that the scar ruptures in 5 per cent of cases; others said it happens in 3 per cent; and several said the risk was 1 per cent. Others did not specify the level of risk. One commented 'No, the risk of rupture is too great. Whilst I might be able to support such a decision it could only be followed through if I was available 24 hours a day'. Just under half (48 per cent) said they would 'allow' a 'trial of labour', albeit with reservations. One in six (14.7 per cent) said they would advise another caesarean, some strongly, but if the woman was 'adamant', 'insistent', 'very keen' they would support her decision. One commented that 'it is possible for non-recurrent obstetric problems and if staff are experienced and supportive, which in the main they tend not to be'. Various observations were made by the majority willing to consider a vaginal birth. One commented 'ideally she should have a caesarean again, but I have supported (successfully) a VBAC after two previous caesareans'. A further 15.3 per cent said it depended on the history. One said 'if two caesareans for non-recurrent cause, Yes; if two for FTP or CPD, No'. Other supportive positions were:

'I would advise her it is a safe thing to do but we would have a low threshold for repeat caesarean.'

'As long as there is no absolute obstetric indication the patient has the choice. There is no evidence that it is unsafe.'

'I would review previous decisions for caesareans, advise on the possibility of risk of scar rupture and support her decision after full discussion.'

'We would advise her that it is safer to have a repeat caesarean but we would support a woman if she wished a trial of labour.'

'She would be allowed a vaginal delivery if: 1) She has laboured before, 2) She wants spontaneous labour, and 3) She accepts the risks.'

'I would discuss the possible risks and document these in detail, discuss the possibility with fellow colleagues and support the patient.'

'I am not against it. I tell them there is a 1 per cent risk of scar rupture.'[79]

Thus, finding supportive professionals may be one of your biggest hurdles.

VBAC at home (often abbreviated to HBAC – home birth after caesarean)

The 1994 study of home births compared low-risk women who had booked for home birth with those booked for hospital birth. The home birth group had fewer interventions in labour, and although some were transferred because of slow progress, the caesarean section and assisted vaginal birth rate was half that of those booked for hospital birth. The outcome for the babies was similar and the NICE guidelines for caesarean section say that women should be told that their risk of having a caesarean is halved if they book for a home birth.[80]

Even if you do have to transfer to hospital, the further along you are in your labour when you enter hospital, the more likely you are to have a vaginal birth. It is also recorded that in hospital one type of intervention leads to another and often culminates in caesarean section.[81] Thus by planning a home birth, you can retain a degree of control over what happens to you and labour in as natural a way as possible. Whether or not it is 'safer' for women planning VBAC to plan a home birth or not is uncertain. As the evidence given above shows, overall VBAC leads to better outcomes for you and your baby than planned repeat caesareans. But most of this evidence comes from studies conducted in hospitals. What this means is that your choice to give birth at home is a personal one and one that you will have to make once you have collected all the relevant information about your previous caesarean, your current pregnancy and the support you will need.

What you have to decide is whether you would be able to face a bad outcome for the baby if you are the one woman in a thousand who does have a scar dehiscence which cannot be dealt with immediately at home. By the time you transfer to hospital the scar may have given way completely and the baby expelled into the abdominal cavity. When the placenta separates then the baby will die. The evidence from many women collected by the VBAC information and advice groups is that hundreds of women have had VBACs at home without any babies dying. It may be that the one in 1,000 figure is too high as at home there are no interventions but there is still a small risk of the scar becoming unzipped. The home birth website has useful information that could help you to make your decision (see www.homebirth.org.uk/vbachome.htm).

One of the women who gave their VBAC stories for this book, Amanda, is now training to be a midwife and recently she told us 'as I learn more, my VBAC story is more of a warning to avoid hospitals and stay at home! I strongly feel that a lot of the problems could have been avoided if I had trusted my own instincts and not succumbed to the medical mode of VBAC'. (See Amanda's story on page 45.)

Another of our VBAC mothers, Clair, had planned a home birth for her second child after the caesarean birth of her first. She told us how the transfer to hospital at the insistence of the midwives led to her abandoning her VBAC plans and a second caesarean:

When I was pregnant with my second child I planned a home water birth with NHS midwives. I had a struggle to get this arranged but in the end they agreed. I'm still not sure of the reason for my second caesarean section, my notes say delay in second stage but there was never any concern over me or the baby. I went into spontaneous labour, my waters broke and my contractions were strong and regular. The midwives were called but when they gave me a VE I lost a small blood clot. I was 4cm dilated. After a second VE I lost a little more blood and the midwife strongly urged me to transfer to hospital, I was 7cm dilated. I agreed. From then on it was a cascade of intervention. The bleeding stopped but I was told I had to be strapped to monitors, a scalp clip was fitted to my baby's head and a drip was put in my hand. I found out later that my notes were marked as FTP as I stuck at 8cm for about an hour after I transferred in but the consultant allowed me a little more time. I reached fully dilated but had a 45 minutes 'rest and be thankful' stage which the doctor was worried about. My contractions started again and I had a strong urge to push but I was then flat on my back and I couldn't get back up on my own as I was tangled up in all the wires from the monitors and the drip so I was told to stay like that. I was allowed one hour of pushing on my back then the doctor said my baby was stuck and I would have to have a ventouse and if that didn't work a caesarean section. I had no other choice but to agree. I was told I had to have an epidural for the ventouse but it was too strong so I could no longer feel to push. As a result the ventouse failed and they performed the CS.

I have spoken about my experience to a couple of midwives and whilst they did not witness my labour they said that the bleeding was most likely a bloody show or cervical erosion and that if I had stayed at home I probably could have delivered my daughter vaginally without any problems. I think the intervention of the ventouse was down to the impatience of the doctor as I did not deliver my baby in the one hour allowed for the second stage in women attempting a VBAC. Once the epidural was in and the ventouse failed there was no option but to perform the CS.

Another woman who contacted us, Heather, had a successful VBAC after a caesarean for her first baby following failure to progress and fetal distress. She chose a hospital VBAC because she wanted to exercise control and choice over which hospital she went to rather than starting a home birth and being transferred to the local hospital. She would have preferred an HBAC. She told us:

I had a VBAC in hospital in January (2006), following one prior section. There's not really much of a story – I turned up and pushed him out about 15 minutes later (he was 10lb 4oz). I ended up going to hospital because I didn't trust the community midwives not to transfer me and I wanted to pick a less interventionist hospital than the nearest one. I sometimes feel I've missed out by not having a home birth.

Even though I had the non-interventionist birth I'd planned (and discussed with the Supervisor of Midwives) I feel it was mainly down to luck and turning up at the hospital ready to push. It wasn't deliberately planned that way – I think the journey was about three-quarters of an hour – but it did mean I didn't have to argue about no monitoring and no timescales. The midwife who 'collected' me from the waiting room (my husband had helped me in and then had to move the car to the car-park) was trying to take me into the admissions room (where they assess and monitor) and only changed her mind when I got on all fours, moaned and announced loudly that I was about to poo! My only examination was when they pulled my trousers off and announced that the head was well down.

I don't think there was a lot of benefit to being in hospital, and I'd endured an incredibly uncomfortable journey. I did have stitches for a second-degree tear – I don't know if these could have been done at home, but I also feel I pushed too hard as I was quite stressed at that point. Possibly at home I would have been calmer and been able to push him out more gently. The time at home had been very relaxed, contractions started during an evening antenatal yoga class, and had built up slowly. It was very peaceful with me leaning on my birth ball and my husband playing on the PC and watching football (you can watch football through the night on Channel 5 apparently!), there if I needed a drink or a snack but otherwise just letting me get on with it.

Some health professionals believe that the perceived 'risks' associated with VBAC are too high to advise women to have a home birth and that VBAC should only be performed in hospitals equipped to care for women at high risk (i.e. capacity to respond to acute obstetric emergencies)[82,83,84,85] and that home birth is not recommended.[86] We do not agree as women are capable of making up their own minds about the risk–benefit ratio of their course of action. There are no randomised controlled trials of VBAC at home versus hospital and these are unlikely to be done.

We are not aware of any studies on the relative success of VBAC comparing home and hospital births. Some women can be affected by being in hospital (white coat syndrome) which makes them more anxious and therefore affects the progress of labour leading to the labour being diagnosed as taking too long (dystocia or failure to progress) which can ultimately lead to caesarean section.

In a major survey of home births conducted in 1994, 53 of the women giving birth at home had previous caesareans, 38 (72 per cent) of whom had successful HBAC. The other 15 women were transferred to hospital but the report does not state whether they achieved VBAC or had another caesarean. Although the number of women in this study with previous caesareans was relatively small, it does show that the majority of those women who planned an HBAC achieved it.[87]

Of the seven women who gave their VBAC stories or shared their experiences with us for this book, three were home births and four in hospital. We do not mean to suggest that a large proportion of VBACs occur at home as we know the home birth rate generally is only around 2 per cent. However, the stories give us faith that HBAC is a safe and viable option for women who choose it. Of our HBAC stories, two women (Clair and Taryn) had two previous caesareans and another (Nikki) had four. So we know that HBAC is not only possible after one caesarean but also after a number of previous caesareans. However, an important point to raise is that all three women in these HBAC stories employed independent midwives. We are not suggesting that this is the key to successful HBAC but rather that for women who can afford this option, it appears to produce good results.

The key to successful VBAC is finding supportive health professionals whether you go with care from the National Health Service (NHS) or choose to employ an independent midwife with back-up support from NHS services.

Getting support from NHS midwives

Home births are usually attended by community midwives. To book a home birth you will need to contact the Head of Midwifery or Supervisor of Midwives at your local hospital. You do not need the support of your GP, in fact you do not have to discuss it with your GP unless you want to.

You may need to negotiate with your Health Authority in order get the professional support you need. Women in the UK have a right to home birth but it appears that there is no obligation on the part of the health authority to provide obstetric care at home. Health authorities may be unsupportive of HBAC because of the perceived 'risks', but armed with information and knowledge about the safety of VBAC you should be able to negotiate appropriate care. (See the home birth website for more information and advice on www.homebirth.org.uk/homebirthuk.htm).

One of the mothers who gave her VBAC story for this book, Clair, told us how she struggled to get the agreement of her consultant and midwives for her choice:

> When I found out I was pregnant with my second child I went to see my doctor and I asked him if I had to have my baby in hospital and he said yes. At my booking appointment I asked my midwife if I had to have my baby in hospital and she said yes too. I mentioned I would have liked to have the baby at home and she shook her head. I telephoned AIMS and they gave me a lot of advice and support. They told me it was possible to have a home VBAC.

> At my first consultant appointment I told the midwife in the clinic that I wanted to have a home birth. She told me the hospital antenatal clinic was not the place to discuss it. She said she would tell the Head of Midwifery and get her to talk to me about it and that I wasn't to say anything to the consultant because he wouldn't like it. The registrar examined me and brought in the consultant who looked at my previous notes and said he

didn't see why I couldn't have a natural delivery this time as my previous section was for breech presentation. I didn't mention my plans for a home birth.

An appointment was made for me to visit the hospital's labour ward and meet with the Supervisor of Midwifery and my own midwife. They showed me around the labour ward which had recently been refurbished and they showed me the birth pool. I think the point of the visit was to show me how nice the hospital was now and to get me to agree to a hospital birth. They were quite surprised that I still wanted a home birth. They warned me about all the dangers, uterine rupture, bleeding etc. I told them I knew about the risks, I had done a lot of reading and I still wanted a home birth. They were concerned about getting me to hospital in an emergency but I live a five-minute drive from the hospital and five minutes from the local ambulance station so I didn't see it being too much of a problem. They said that it would be hard to get me into the car if there was an emergency and that the ambulances aren't always at the ambulance station and it could take 20 minutes for one to get to me. They said they would have to put an ambulance on standby when I went into labour just in case.

There were a lot of conditions put on my home birth. I would have to go to hospital if I went into labour before 37 weeks or after 41 weeks, if there was any bleeding, if there was any meconium (a sign of fetal distress), if my temperature or blood pressure went up or if no midwives were available to come out to me

My midwife wrote absolutely everything down in my notes but it wasn't until my overdue consultant appointment at 40 + 4 weeks that the registrar noticed that I was booked for a 'home confinement'. He almost fell off his chair when I told him and he discharged me from consultant care in disgust. Later that day I got a phone call from one of the midwives asking me to go back and see the consultant to talk about my plans but I refused as I said it would change nothing. I knew of all the risks and I was happy to stay at home.

It was quite a traumatic pregnancy, I felt that I had to fight everyone to get what I wanted. If I hadn't had the support of AIMS, the homebirth.org website and the people on the ukhomebirth and ukvbachbac Yahoo groups I would have accepted what my midwife and doctor had told me, that I would have to have my baby in hospital.

In a recent statement on home birth from the Nursing and Midwifery Council, the Chief Executive, Sarah Thewlis, stated:

...all midwives have a responsibility to ensure that all women receive care that is based on partnership with women and respects the individuality of a woman and her family. Women have the right to make their own decisions on these issues if they are competent to do so and midwives have a duty of care to respect a woman's choice.[88]

Where a midwife does not feel confident to attend a home birth it is unacceptable for her to refuse a home birth and take no further action. Rather the midwifery guidelines state that she must take steps to update her knowledge and experience to ensure her confidence with home birth in the future and, importantly, refer you on to another midwife who does have the confidence to attend a home birth.

Employing an independent midwife

Independent midwives (IM) are fully trained and qualified midwives who have chosen to work outside of the NHS and are self-employed. As such they can be engaged by individuals to work with and for them. The going rate for an IM is from about £1,800 to £4,500 (approximately) for the whole package of care. You are still entitled to NHS treatment and services such as blood tests and scans if you employ an IM.

The IM's role is to care for you during pregnancy, birth and afterwards. They can work with you whether you are planning a home birth or a hospital birth. If you start labour at home and transfer to hospital they can accompany you as your birth partner or supporter but would be unable to give clinical care once in hospital except in a tiny minority of cases so your clinical care would transfer to NHS staff at this stage.

The advantage of having an IM is that you can choose your midwife and be assured of continuity of care. IMs are supportive of women's choices and many take on the care of women who are deemed 'high risk' including those who have had previous caesareans. They give you advice and information to empower you to make informed decisions about the birth of your baby. They will be there to support you during labour and act as your advocate in terms of ensuring your wishes are considered at times when you may not be able to assert yourself. You will see from the birth stories in this book that the three women who gave birth at home employed IMs although we are not suggesting that this is the only way to achieve an HBAC.

Summary

The fact that a second labour is usually more efficient than the first, and that the weight and position of the baby may be different, all point towards the best option being to aim to give birth vaginally. Obviously, if you had a difficult labour with your previous pregnancy, possibly because of poor management, you may feel that you do not want to plan a VBAC; but given a supportive team of health care professionals who are approachable and available, you may be able to see the benefit of this. In any case, planning to labour rather than planning a repeat caesarean has advantages. First, it is good for the baby to have some squeezing from contractions prior to birth. Second, the lower part of the uterus becomes thinner during labour so even if you do end up with a repeat caesarean, having had some labour may make the operation easier.

It appears from the studies we have looked at and the women we have spoken to that most women value the support to choose vaginal birth regardless of outcome[89] and women who have experienced both vaginal birth and caesarean section are more satisfied with vaginal birth.[90] What you require from your health care professionals when weighing up the pros and cons of VBAC is information and/or counselling which is individualised to you, your past medical history and current situation and includes details of both the short- and long-term benefits and risks.

There is a great deal of debate and a certain amount of concern about VBAC within the medical profession. The birth stories below show that the medical attitudes to individual pregnancies have left many women feeling that they have to do battle with the profession rather than work with it. These examples show that some obstetricians have been seen to make cutting and unhelpful comments, and can be obstructive. This is unfortunate. Childbirth is a very significant event in parents' lives and it is of the utmost importance that the quality of care you receive, both physical and emotional, is of the highest order. Only then will you have good memories of your baby's birth; and when each birthday of your child arrives, you can think back warmly to the important occasion and the support and help you received from those attending the birth.

What you need to know

• *The reason for your previous caesarean(s)*

In the UK you are more likely to find support for your choice of VBAC when your caesarean was done for a reason which is unlikely to recur in your next pregnancy, such as breech presentation or because your labour was taking too long. If the operation was done because it was thought that your labour was taking too long due to your baby being too big to pass through your pelvis, most consultants would advise a repeat caesarean. However, one study showed that even when the first caesarean was done because the baby was thought to be too big, 20 per cent of women gave birth vaginally.[91]

• *The VBAC success rate of the hospital and, preferably, the consultant treating you*

If you plan to give birth in hospital, take your time over choosing your hospital and/or your consultant and do not be rushed into a hasty decision. Assessment of information at a local level will be of more use to you than the results of studies where the skills of hospital staff and the organisation of services may differ significantly from your local unit. Unfortunately the VBAC rates for each hospital are not published so you will need to ask the Head of Midwifery or Midwifery Supervisor at your local unit for this information. If you find that their VBAC rate is low or they are unsupportive of VBAC generally, ask to be assigned to another consultant or find another hospital. Overall caesarean rates are published for each hospital so this may be an indication of attitude towards VBAC. On a very general level, the higher the caesarean rate for a hospital the less likely it is that they are supportive of VBAC. See our book *Caesarean Birth in Britain* (2006) for a list of hospital caesarean rates or look on www.birthchoiceuk.com for more recent information.

• *Hospital policy*

If you plan to give birth in hospital, find out the maternity department's policies regarding the factors that may adversely affect your chances of achieving a VBAC detailed under 'Success of VBAC' on page 12 above and including:

• Continuous electronic fetal monitoring or internal monitoring
• Restriction of food and fluid intake
• Restriction on your ability to move around

- Time limits
- Staff changes
- Acceleration of labour by ARM (artificial rupture of the membranes)
- Induction or augmentation (acceleration of labour with oxytocin)
- Requiring you to go into hospital early in labour
- Use of pain control especially epidural.

In addition:

- If you decide to change hospital from the previous time, ensure that your notes are obtained, together with the results of any X-rays taken after the caesarean.

- Prepare yourself mentally and physically for a VBAC – you've taken a good step towards this by reading this book!

- Contact one of the VBAC support organisations for help and advice, and talk to women who have succeeded with VBAC. This could also help you to decide on which hospital to use or the most supportive health professionals to talk to. See details on pages 97–8.

Birth stories

We have included seven VBAC stories in this section of the book: four took place in hospital and three at home, one after four caesareans! The stories are personal accounts, mostly of positive experiences but also some difficult ones. We hope that sharing these women's emotions and experiences will give you information, hope and determination in choosing VBAC if it is the right option for you.

A positive experience and successful VBAC in hospital

Rachel researched the risks and benefits surrounding VBAC to decide what the best option for her was. She received good support from health care professionals and succeeded with a VBAC in 2004. She told us *I am awestruck at my body's ability to give birth all on its own; my VBAC is the most fulfilling experience of my life.*

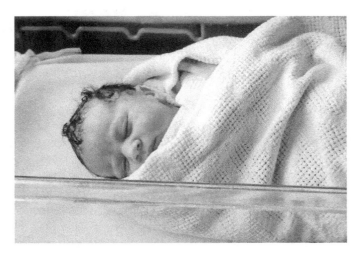

Rachel's VBAC baby Isaac, minutes after his birth

Rachel's VBAC story – Isaac

My first child was born in August 2001 by an elective caesarean section (CS). My pregnancy had gone swimmingly until my 36-week check when the doctor thought that the baby was breech. A scan two days later showed that she was in fact transverse, and the consultant terrified me with talk of a prolapsed cord, and made me stay in hospital. It transpired that in fact she had an unstable lie, and flitted about all over the place, but very rarely head down. I found the situation so stressful, and with little apparent prospect of a natural delivery, that after a week in hospital I asked for a caesarean. Physically this went quite smoothly, but I was unprepared for the psychological impact; subconsciously, I felt that since I had handed over responsibility for her birth to someone else, someone else was also responsible for her care. I didn't have a problem bonding with her, but I struggled to feel that I had the right and the ability to look after her.

Later on I realised that I felt a huge loss at having been unable to experience labour and birth. I think I might not have felt so bad about it if I'd been convinced that a caesarean was unavoidable – If I'd had the chance to labour and it hadn't worked out or if she had still been transverse when I went into labour. With hindsight I felt that I should have waited to go into labour naturally, at which point she might have got into position; if I'd had more support and encouragement rather than all the scaremongering, this might have been an option. I went round looking enviously at all the women I knew who'd had natural deliveries, and even those who'd had an emergency CS since at least they'd had a chance to labour.

Anyway, second time around I was determined to do everything I could to get a natural delivery. I'd seen lots of 'real birth' programmes on TV and they filled me with horror – the poor mum, flat on her back surrounded by medical equipment and doctors telling her what to do. I really wanted and needed this birth to be my experience, not a medical event. I also didn't want to be treated like a ticking time bomb – a rupture waiting to happen. I did lots of reading and decided that medical intervention such as monitoring was unlikely to be of benefit. I did consider a home birth, but I didn't feel confident about it without a confident midwife (which to my mind really meant an independent midwife) so I kept that as a last resort. I was also concerned that this baby would have trouble engaging, given the unstable lie I'd had first time around.

Given that a hospital birth was my most likely outcome, I decided it would be better to get a buy-in from the medical establishment at an early stage rather than wait until I was in labour, and run the risk of being pressurised to change my mind. I met with a registrar, who didn't mind me having a VBAC although she wasn't exactly encouraging. Hospital policy wasn't as bad as I had feared; there was no time limit on labour but she was very unhappy that I refused to have continuous monitoring and was dismissive of other ways of detecting uterine rupture such as monitoring blood pressure and pulse. I went away somewhat discouraged but still determined that I would do things my way. I had lots of lengthy chats with my community midwife about what I wanted (apologies to anyone who ever had an appointment after me!) and after some initial doubts she obviously decided that I really meant it and was very supportive. She arranged for me to see the consultant midwife, who was absolutely fantastic; her attitude was that if that's what I wanted, that's what I would get; no continuous monitoring, no drip, no time limits, no pain relief unless I asked for it, no ban on food and drink. We would plan for a successful natural labour. She wrote a letter to the midwifery staff, and put a copy in my notes explaining this so that I wouldn't get any hassle when the time came. She only asked that I have regular checks with a hand-held Sonicaid and an internal exam every three hours once I was in established labour to make sure that things were progressing. My community midwife also switched me to a different consultant, whose only concern was to have me in for regular checks if I got to 42 weeks. It just goes to show how different they can be!

The only snag at this stage (about 34 weeks) was that the baby was, yes, transverse! The consultant midwife gave me some tips on getting it to turn, which meant that I spent a week in the height of summer with a sarong strapped tightly around my tummy. The baby must have found this as uncomfortable as I did, because a week later he was head down and he stayed put.

The great day came when, just before midnight two days before my due date, my waters broke. Having called our friend to take care of our daughter, we duly trotted off to hospital. They confirmed that the waters had indeed gone, but the baby wasn't engaged and I wasn't dilated at all yet. On account of the lack of engagement and the previous caesarean, they were keen for us to stay in hospital, but as I was only having contractions every ten minutes and we felt that nothing would happen for ages we declined and went home. They didn't pressurise us about this decision which I felt was down to the fact that they could see from my notes that I had given my birth a great deal of thought. We arrived home at 2.30am and I sent my husband to bed to get some rest. This proved to be a bad idea because my contractions instantly speeded up to five minutes apart and, on my own, I struggled to cope. An hour later, at 3.30am, I woke him up and suggested that we return to hospital, so back we went. They did an internal examination at 4.30am and I was devastated to learn that I was only 1cm dilated, as I was finding it really hard to cope. Ironically, now that I wanted to stay, they were keen for us to go back home, or at least down to the ward to walk about. Fortunately they didn't press the point and instead offered me gas and air and a warm bath. So much for my resolve to have no pain relief – I didn't know anything could hurt so much! The next few hours were a bit of a blur. Since I wasn't, in their view, in established labour, I didn't get the 15-minute checks (I think they stopped by a couple of times). I was left in my husband's rather overwhelmed hands. Eventually I felt that I couldn't cope any more and sent my husband off to find a midwife and demand pethidine. The logical part of my brain knew that actually this probably wouldn't help at all, since the contractions were more or less continuous, but I was pretty desperate by now. I was even having fond thoughts of the caesarean! A midwife finally showed up and talked me through some contractions, which really helped. She opined that I was probably 3–4cm dilated, which left me feeling that I really couldn't cope with another five hours of this. She asked me to get out of the bath so that she could check what was going on and we could make a new plan; this took some time as I was waiting for a gap in the contractions before I moved, but there never was a gap – just a variation from very painful to excruciatingly painful.

I finally made it onto a bed at 8am and was heartened to find that actually I was 8cm dilated. At this point my husband went off to go to the toilet, the midwife wandered off to find someone else and I found that I couldn't breathe. When this happened a second time it dawned on me that this was probably what pushing was, so I told the midwife when she reappeared. Another contraction and I could feel something, so I told the midwife and she had another look, at which point it was all systems go – the baby was coming very soon! My husband asked what did that mean – in the next ten minutes or so? No – it meant in the next minute! Another contraction, and out popped Isaac at 8.14am weighing 7lb 15oz. So the notes read: Stage 1: 3½ hours (actually time from 1cm to 8cm), Stage 2: 14 minutes (actually 8cm to delivery). The fly in the ointment was that the speed of the second stage meant that I tore really badly, and had to go into theatre to be stitched up under a spinal block. There was a bit of déjà vu – same place my daughter was delivered, drips, etc., but frankly I didn't care at this stage. I was just glad it was over and I'd done it!

I don't regret not trying for an HBAC, although if I were to have another child I would do so; once labour got going I was fairly oblivious to my surroundings. The only thing I would have changed would have been to have a doula as a bit more support would have made a big difference, and might have enabled me to avoid tearing so badly. I am also aware that I was lucky that labour progressed so quickly that there was no need for anyone to even think about intervention; if things had gone slowly then I wonder if there might have been some pressure to intervene regardless of my birth plan. I'm still really thrilled that I did it, but also sad that I didn't trust my body enough to do so first time around.

STORY TWO

A difficult VBAC in hospital

Amanda had a successful vaginal (ventouse) birth of her second child six years after a caesarean birth. The vaginal birth was quite traumatic with some complications but Amanda was glad she persisted and would choose VBAC again. She told us *I still feel chuffed with myself for achieving a VBAC as I was told I was not a good candidate.*

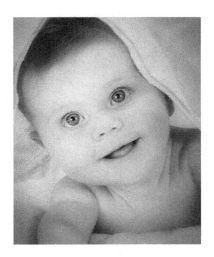

Amanda's VBAC baby, Lucy

Amanda's VBAC story – Lucy Victoria

My obstetric history is by no means unusual. My first pregnancy progressed well – although I did have glucose in my urine on quite a few occasions, but had a tolerance test which came out ok. Labour was induced at ten days over and I eventually had an emergency caesarean after three attempts at induction had failed. On day 13, after rupturing membranes achieved its aim, I 'failed to progress' further than 9cm. Emily Louise was born weighing in at 9lb 5oz. At the time I felt I had saved either my or my baby's life by having this caesarean but to find 'failure' written on most of my notes came as a shock as I had no idea that I had been against the clock. From this point I was informed by most medical staff that if I was to have more children then I would of course be having an elective caesarean. This put me off – as I didn't recover well from the first – until I read about VBAC. Six years later I gave birth to Lucy Victoria but, although I got my VBAC, it wasn't without problems. If you are planning a VBAC because it will be easier than a CS and recovery will be quicker then do not read my story; but if you want to feel a baby being born the way it was supposed to be and you want to feel your body doing this wondrous thing called labour then yes, VBAC will be for you.

My community midwife was never anything but supportive. I had told her about my first birth as there was nothing in writing as I had delivered in Germany (Forces). I knew the problem was to do with my baby's size, a maternity nurse had told me this afterwards as Emily had 'got stuck' – she had told me this in broken English. Because of the CS I was under the consultant and attended my first appointment at 24 weeks. I had asked about the possibility of using the birthing pool, but of course this was not allowed. I told the registrar of my concerns about baby's size as again I showed glucose in urine regularly throughout this pregnancy also. He booked me for a scan at 34 weeks to estimate the size and to talk about options available to me then.

At 34 weeks I met my consultant and had my scan which estimated my baby's size at 6lb 10oz. My consultant told me this was only borderline large, and the size of the baby was not really the issue as the estimation could be as much as 15 per cent out. I had asked if I could be induced at 39 weeks to give me the best chance of a vaginal birth with a smaller baby. I was told in no uncertain terms that because of my scar the only way I could try for a VBAC was if I spontaneously laboured as I was far too high risk for inducement and anyway who would want to be induced at 39 weeks? I had got really upset as he had indicated that I really should consider an elective caesarean section and he was quite prepared to do this at 39 weeks if I wanted. His support culminated in telling me that he had had only two maternal deaths in his career and both were from ruptured scars. I went home very upset as at no point had anybody indicated that I was such a high risk. That night I hit the Internet and found some very interesting facts from a website called 'Radical Midwives' which then led me to the VBAC information and support group. I telephoned and had a wonderful chat with one of their members. She also sent me loads of information, her own personal stories and the name of the Radical Midwife for my area. This gave me the confidence to carry on with my own VBAC as I was on the verge of saying to hell with it and just do the caesarean and get it over with. Why on earth should I want to put myself through this stress when there was such an easy way out? I also called my community midwife who came for a home visit and went through the options again.

At 36 weeks I went back to see my consultant, this time armed with reports, tables, statistics and a lot of confidence! I told him he had treated me like a walking scar and that the information he had given me was misleading. We managed to thrash out a compromise. He was not willing to discuss the issue of baby's size and my worries on this issue as he said it was not relevant but let me have membrane sweeps and as long as I spontaneously laboured I had a reasonable chance. I wasn't happy as I didn't spontaneously labour first time, drip and gel had also failed – only ARM had worked. I could however try raspberry leaf, sex, and any other remedies within reason. At least I had got something. At 37 weeks I began having contractions, 5–7 minutes apart, I went up to the hospital to have them checked out, and yes, I was 1–2cm but was sent home as it was latent first stage and could go on for hours. In fact it went on and off for four weeks.

At 38 weeks I saw the consultant, still in a lot of discomfort, no change. 'See you again at 40 weeks.'

Before I attended my consultant appointment I telephoned the consultant unit to ask for advice on what was likely to be discussed at the next appointment and could I ask for a membrane sweep and what it entails etc. Sadly, the midwife I spoke to wasn't at all co-operative and told me in no uncertain terms to attend the appointment and it would all be explained there. I felt that she couldn't possibly tell me information that went against consultant advice. I then telephoned the midwife recommended by the VBAC support group, who rang me back that evening and went through everything and explained in detail.

At 40 weeks + 3 days, I saw the midwife at the consultant unit and asked for a membrane sweep. She wasn't convinced it would do any good until closer to 41 weeks but I persisted. She did it and also booked me in for another sweep at 41 weeks and an inducement at 41 + 3 days. It was all happening exactly the same as first time, and all I could see was caesarean. I spent a day sobbing. I knew I wasn't going to spontaneously labour.

At 41 weeks I went back to the hospital to have my membranes swept again. Although my contractions had increased in intensity they were still only 7–10 minutes apart and would fade away. My membranes were swept again and I was left on the fetal monitor for half an hour just for precaution. It was here that I felt rather damp below, and on checking I had left a rather large damp patch, but it could not be decided if my waters had been broken or just grazed. I couldn't now go back home so I was admitted to the ward to be checked again in the morning. I had a more uncomfortable night as my contractions were significantly more intense but I still did not think my waters were broken.

The next morning I met the consultant on duty, she asked me what I wanted to do, so I told her I wanted my waters broken and see if that set me off in established labour. She agreed and booked me in for 10.30am. No problems.

My waters were broken at 10.30am where a very small amount of meconium was found, and within an hour or so I was in established labour with TENS attached.
I am afraid time is sort of hazy but it was around 12–1pm that the pain got really intense and I tried the gas and air. It made me sick but I carried on using it with Marilyn Manson and Linkin Park on the MP3 player we had brought

in. By 2pm (ish) I needed something else and wanted an epidural. However, on checking, I was 8–9cm dilated and my midwife Donna thought it would not be a good idea as I didn't have long to go, but I could have pethidine. I did and I was sick again! It was 4pm and pain was now getting unbearable so I again asked for an epidural. I was checked again and I was still 9cm; my midwife went to ask about one. Unfortunately the anaesthetist was in theatre and would be at least 45 minutes but would come to me next. The contractions were incredibly intense and I tried to get myself comfortable but being stuck on the bed and constantly monitored inhibited my movements and the insistence of a cannula in situ in case of an emergency was restrictive. I pulled it out eventually as it kept catching.

At 5pm I was ready to push, but I had a rim of cervix, and the baby was unable to come down. I couldn't stop the urge to push and was sick again. The consultant came to check me and found that when I did push she was able to push back the rim of cervix and baby was able to come down. She said she wanted to try and pull her out with a ventouse in theatre and if that failed I was set up for a caesarean. By now I had been pushing for over an hour and was completely knackered. I had somehow got into my head that it would be another hour of pushing in theatre. Donna reassured me it would be two or three pushes maximum. If it failed then it would be a section. I was set up in stirrups, local anaesthetics inside and around the vaginal area, a theatre full of people. A midwife on each leg, one on left shoulder and hubby on right shoulder, a registrar and consultant with ventouse cap at the ready. The contraction came and I pushed for all I was worth. The consultant asked if I wanted to feel the baby's head. I was expecting a bit of head but in fact I stuck my finger up my baby's nose as the whole head was out and facing up! The second push took almost seven minutes as my baby's shoulder was stuck. Eventually she was out and Donna placed her on my stomach, we made a quick eye contact, and she promptly weed on me! We had had a little girl – Lucy Victoria born at 18.39 hours on 19 October 2003, weighing in at 9lb 3oz.

Unfortunately Lucy didn't breathe very well and was whisked away for extra help. It did improve and her breathing was fine but she was traumatised from the birth and was taken to the Special Care Baby Unit. It took 45 minutes to sew me up, followed by three hours in recovery on a drip as my uterus was not contracting down as it should.

I got to see Lucy in her incubator at about 10pm where I found out she had a fractured clavicle from shoulder dystocia, left-arm palsy and a sore and swollen head. Although she had weed on me at delivery, she had not weed for her first night so was being treated for renal failure also. I had suffered a major tear and episiotomy. After visiting Lucy in special baby care I returned to the ward (in a wheelchair) and tried to get to sleep – it was about 11.30pm. The pain in my right bum cheek was immense so I called the midwife to ask about some more pain relief. She came and checked me out and told me she was going to call the doctor as the bruising and swelling was pretty severe. The pain relief did not work, the pain was more intense and still no doctor at 12.30am. I called the midwife on at least two more occasions, finally I had to put my TENS machine on my bum cheek and I was clawing the walls! Doctor came at about 1.30am and I was taken back into the labour ward to be checked. I was seen by the duty consultant who advised conservative treatment which was to 'wait and see'. He didn't want to open everything back up unless it was absolutely necessary. I got a pethidine injection and was asleep by 2.15am and wheeled back to the ward. As long as the pain relief was given I was able to cope but my bum cheek was solid, black and very uncomfortable!

Although I was able to drive my car after two weeks it took over ten weeks to recover from this birth which included a severe bout of anaemia. VBAC, would I do it again? You bet! And it just goes to show you can VBAC a traumatic ventouse delivery with no problems for the scar, without spontaneously labouring. I look back now and feel desperately robbed of the vaginal birth I had planned for my first. Both labours from breaking of waters were identical: quick progress to 9cm, anterior lip of cervix and a baby in a difficult position to birth (direct OP), which is back to back with mother, yet one ends in a caesarean and one in a vaginal birth. Hindsight is a wonderful thing and I often wonder what would have happened if I had been 'allowed' to labour in water, for instance, or to birth at home in familiar surroundings with no time constraints. To let my body have the freedom to dictate the proceedings and not hospital protocols. If there were a next time it would be in water, at home and with me in full control.

STORY THREE

A distressing VBAC in hospital

Tina had three caesareans before she realised that VBAC was an option. She had to change consultants three times before finding one who would support her.

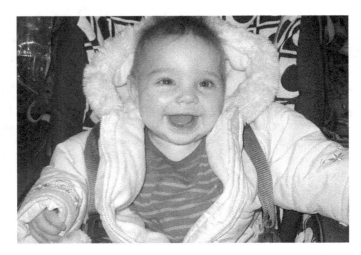

Tina's VBA3C baby, Lydia

Tina's VBA3C story – Lydia

My first baby, Mitchell, was born in 1987 by emergency caesarean section (CS). I was induced at 35 weeks for severe pre-eclampsia and had the caesarean for FTP and FD. My second child, Florence, was born in 2000 and I was talked out of VBAC by my consultant, although with hindsight there was no good reason why I couldn't have had a very straightforward VBAC. My third child, Madeleine was born in 2003. She was breech all the way through the pregnancy and I didn't know that VBAC would even have been possible so was just booked in for an elective CS.

It was only when I had a look on the Internet to see how many caesareans you are 'allowed' to have that I found out VBAC might be an option if I conceived again. I got pregnant soon after and just assumed that no-one would have a problem with my requesting a VBAC. How wrong can you be? I ended up changing my consultant three times before finding one who would support me (the last time at 37 weeks). Again, I didn't realise that I could have insisted on midwifery care only until it was too late, but I'll know for next time!

I awoke on the sofa at 6am on Sunday 23 April, my due date, feeling a little odd. I wasn't quite sure what had woken me; I just knew that something was happening. (I had been sleeping on the sofa for a few nights as I had finally reached the point of hugeness where I couldn't even get on and off our high bed!) I lay there for a while, pondering. By 6.45am I realised that I was in labour. I had been having strong, regular Braxton Hicks for three or four weeks, for at least a couple of hours at a time, but always in the evenings. This was the first time I had ever had contractions of any kind first thing in the morning, and they felt completely different from any that I had felt before – rather than tightenings – these were unmistakeably labour pains. People had always told me that I would just know when I was in labour, and they were right.

Everyone else in the house was still asleep, and I stayed where I was, hugging my secret to myself until they started to appear. I heard my husband, Peter, get up to the girls at about 8am, and hoped that they'd come down, but no, they did their usual trick and climbed into our big bed for a bit of morning

TV. I debated going upstairs to tell Peter the news, but decided it was much too far away and would involve far too much effort, so I stayed where I was. They finally appeared at 9am. I told Peter that I had been having contractions every 15 minutes since I'd woken up and that this was it. I think I surprised him a little by how calm I was. He said he wouldn't bother taking the girls to Mass that morning, but I insisted that I was fine as long as they came straight back afterwards. I think I stayed where I was until about 11am, just before they got back from church. I knew that whilst I had to conserve my energy, I had to balance that with being as active as possible, and I was starting to find lying down rather uncomfortable.

I pottered around the house for a while, had a shower, some breakfast and read the Sunday papers. I texted my doula, Bushra, to tell her that I was in labour but that there was definitely no need to come over yet as I was fine. At 12.30pm I decided to ring the hospital to find out who was on duty that day – a team had been put together for me previously who were all supportive of VBAC and I needed to know that there would be someone familiar there for me when I went in. The Supervisor of Midwives who I had met before wasn't on duty. The sister who had shown us around the unit and introduced us to our fabulous consultant was on annual leave. My consultant was also not in that day either. Brilliant! My community midwife was in Italy until the following day too. My heart was sinking rapidly. The midwife I spoke to on the phone asked who I was, and whether or not I was in labour, and when I told her she immediately put me on hold and went off to find someone. When she came back she told me that they wanted me to come straight in. This was exactly what I didn't want to do so I asked if I could contact a community midwife for an assessment first and then come in later when I was ready. No, she insisted that they wanted me straight in. It was easier to agree, so I said I'd be along presently. As if!

At this point, I thought it might be nice to have a bath as the contractions were getting stronger, so I went and floated in there for a while before getting bored. I rang my mum to let her know that she'd need to come round later on (she arrived about 20 minutes later, bless her, all in a flap) and got Peter to put the TENS machine on. We disappeared into our bedroom at this point and made ourselves a little nest on the bed with the beanbag so that I could get comfortable. My feet had swelled to enormous proportions and my darling husband had spent hours over the last three or four weeks trying to massage them back into shape, and he spent a blissful hour doing the same for me now. I thought it might be a good idea to finish packing my hospital bag as Peter was driving me crackers about it (for some reason), and by 4.30pm I decided that maybe it was time to get ourselves over to the hospital. My contractions were now coming every six or seven minutes and were lasting a good minute and a half.

I came downstairs to find my mum still flapping, my 19-year-old son – who was fortunately not due back at university until the next day – being very calm and my two beautiful daughters, Florence and Madeleine, playing nicely. I had a few tears from Florence when she realised we were leaving for the hospital, but generally we managed to make our escape pretty easily. We can get to Good Hope Hospital in about 15 minutes on the M6 toll road, all very smooth, straight and quick. So my darling husband decided to go the other way. When I asked why we weren't going on the toll road, he informed me that it was Sunday so the traffic would be ok the other way. MISSING THE POINT??!! I'M IN LABOUR HERE!!! For the sake of calm, I only said this in my head and bit my tongue. By the time we were almost there (after hitting every bump on the way) my contractions had speeded up a little to five minutes apart, and I was really pleased as the plan had always been that we wouldn't go in until I had got to that point. I only had to make him stop once over a particularly bumpy bit of road during a contraction, so all in all, it could have been worse.

By the time we got up to the delivery suite, it was almost 5.30pm and the welcoming party were almost wetting themselves – it had only taken me five hours to get there after ringing them! Fair play to them, they almost managed to convey an air of indifference to my lateness, but I would have loved to have been a fly on the wall in the staff room that afternoon! I was shown into the delivery room right next to the staff room and fully expected a barrage of monitoring etc., but the lovely Scottish midwife who had been assigned to me was very relaxed and we had a chat about my birth plan, which she had already read and she suggested that if I wanted to go for a walk first, there was no rush. (I had agreed that they could monitor me for half an hour on arrival so that they could get baseline readings, on the condition that I wasn't strapped down flat on my back.) She asked me if I wanted her to examine me, and I thought it would be a good idea – if I hadn't started to dilate I was going to go back home and wait it out there (although I obviously didn't tell her that!) But guess what: I was already 4cm! I can't tell you how excited I was – my only previous experience of labour was induction for pre-eclampsia at 35 weeks with my son, and after 16 hours of tooth-grindingly hard labour, I never got past 4cm, so this was a real achievement for me; and I have to say that it had been embarrassingly easy this time too. I was quite desperate for some coffee by now and as the hospital café was so awful, we got back in the car and drove into Sutton Coldfield to forage for something decent. Not sure that my midwife had been expecting us to leave the hospital completely, but what the heck! I texted Bushra again to let her know that she could come over to the hospital when she was ready, and to let her know of my fantastic progress.

We got back about half an hour or so later, I unpacked my bag, got monitored and settled myself onto the birthing ball. They brought me a big bean bag in too, but my feet were hurting too much to get comfortable on it. I alternated between the ball and an armchair, on which I found kneeling, holding on to the back, to be the most comfortable position. I had assumed that the intermittent monitoring which I had agreed to would be done by strapping the monitor to me whilst I was sitting up on the ball or the chair but I was pleasantly surprised when I realised that all it involved was my midwife holding it against my tummy for a minute every so often. My midwife asked me if I had received the letter expected from my consultant, written to satisfy the Board and their legal team. As I hadn't received it (it arrived in the next day's post) she read it to me, and seemed very nervous of my reaction to it. It had been very carefully worded but there was nothing in there that I wasn't expecting apart from a paragraph concerning using the birthing pool – it had been decided that they couldn't allow it in case I needed to get out quickly. I was initially quite cross about this as it had been previously agreed that it wouldn't be a problem (and Peter had packed his swimming shorts especially!) My midwife asked if I wanted her to ring my consultant to see if she would change her mind and I said yes. When she left the room, Peter and I discussed it, and I said that whilst I was disappointed, every other thing that I had stipulated in my birth plan had been agreed to so if the answer was no, I would accept it with good grace. The answer was no (of course) but they had no problem with me labouring in the bath if I wanted to. (As it turned out, I would never have had time to get into the pool as you have to be at least 5cm dilated, but more of that later.)

Bushra arrived at about 8.45pm, essential oils and homeopathic remedies at the ready, followed shortly after by the anaesthetist who I had agreed to talk to. I have awful veins, and had agreed to have a cannula in place as long as it wasn't in my hand. For the first time ever, I was actually given a local anaesthetic first before the cannula was put in – luxury! Unfortunately, the anaesthetist couldn't find the vein in my left arm, so he had to start all over again in my right arm. (Again, as it turned out, I made exactly the right decision to have the cannula put in at this stage.) Not long after this, my consultant appeared to say hello (quite impressive I thought, considering it was her day off and quite late by this time on a Sunday evening). She apologised to me regarding the pool issue, and I think if the pressure hadn't been put on her by the legal people, she would have agreed to it. A staff change saw my midwife leave and be replaced by the sister who had shown us around the unit which I was really pleased about. The first midwife was lovely but a familiar face makes such a difference. She asked if I minded a student midwife being present, which I had no problem with. The more VBACs students see the more commonplace it should become in the future.

I was reassessed at 10.30pm and was deeply disappointed to find that I was still only 4cm, still not thinning or effacing and the baby's head was still very high. At no point was any mention made of time limits, for which I was really grateful – it was something I was insistent on in my birth plan. My midwife didn't seem to be at all concerned about my lack of visible progress and she suggested a walk. This time, I restricted myself to the hospital! We walked up and down the stairs a few times and availed ourselves of the dreadful coffee machine. I was feeling slightly queasy by this time, but Peter had been nagging me for hours to eat something so I agreed to the minestrone soup (foolishly). We did a little more sideways stair climbing and returned to my room.

By this time it was around 12.30am and I was feeling fairly tired. My midwife suggested I lay down on my side for a while to see if I could get some sleep and I stupidly agreed. She took the opportunity to put the monitor on so that she could get a good trace while I was lying down. Within what felt like seconds of lying down, my pains changed from being totally manageable to totally unbearable. I had been increasing the intensity of the TENS machine throughout the course of the evening, and by this time it felt as if it was having no effect whatsoever. Peter and Bushra had settled themselves into the armchairs to sleep and I can remember lying there, crying, thinking why aren't they doing something for me? It felt like hours before they came over to me (although I'm sure it wasn't!) and I begged them to help me. I couldn't bear lying down, I felt sick and I was starting to lose control. It was after 2am by this time and as I was in so much pain the medical staff re-examined me only to find that there had still been no change. I couldn't believe it. How could there possibly have been no change? I was in bloody agony! I think it was around this point that I started begging for an epidural. I was as sick as a dog, and then had diarrhoea and I felt awful. Peter remained very calm and kept pointing out to me that I had insisted I didn't want an epidural in my birth plan, and how much I'd regret it if I had one. I was beside myself! But I really really NEED one! How could he be so cruel?

When I look back now, I had all the classic signs of transition, but all I could see was 4cm and hours and hours of pain in front of me. My midwife suggested other forms of pain relief and I turned into a petulant child – I didn't like pethidine, and I didn't like gas and air, so there. They ran me a bath and helped me in – utter bliss. The midwife brought the gas and air in, and hooked it over the side of the bath 'just in case you change your mind!' 'Oh... My God! How fabulous is gas and air??!!' They had turned the lights off and just left the door ajar so it was really dim – just me and the gas and air. I can still remember the first couple of lungfuls – I just lay there for a while afterwards with a silly grin on my face – why hadn't they given me this earlier??!! As the bath had been running, Bushra told me that Michel Odent reckons you can go from 5cm to fully dilated in an hour and a half in water. I just wanted to tell her to f*** off at the time! As if!

I lost all track of time at this point – I vaguely remember Bushra pouring warm water over my belly at one point, and me demanding in words of no more than one syllable that I have more hot water in the bath immediately. If pressed, I'd say that I must have been in there for at least two or three hours but apparently after about half an hour or so, I was heard making 'pushy' noises. I do remember my midwife coming in and asking me if I was pushing. It's odd as I could think perfectly clearly, but I just couldn't find the words to speak properly. I thought to myself 'how can I possibly be pushing? I'm only bloody 4cm dilated!' Five minutes later, she came back in again and said 'you are pushing, aren't you?' I was just about to disagree when I had an almighty contraction and I thought bloody hell, yes I am pushing!

At that point, all hell broke loose. All the lights went on, the bathroom was suddenly full of people, and they were trying to tell me I had to get out of the bath. I don't know if I said it out loud or just in my head but I definitely remember saying 'you have got to be having a f***ing laugh if you think I can get out of this bath now!' To this day, I have no idea quite how they got me out, but the next thing I remember is being on my hands and knees, hanging onto the raised back of the bed for grim death. Again, I lost all concept of time, but it was somewhere between 30 and 45 minutes from this point until Lydia was born. I pushed with all my might and I felt a huge pop and was overjoyed that my baby had been born so easily. To say that I was crushed when they told me it was just my waters going would be an understatement! I do recall saying that I hoped it had got them all! Shortly after this, I decided that there was no way on God's earth I was going to get this baby out without assistance – I had Peter on one side telling me how well I was doing (just told him to shut up), Bushra on the other side telling me what a strong powerful woman I was (just told her to f*** off again, I believe!) and the midwife at the business end telling me I was doing it all by myself perfectly well (yeah, thanks a bunch for the help!)

I had had visions beforehand when planning my birth of how calm and peaceful the delivery room was going to be, how serene and in control I would be, how I'd be listening to my midwife and pushing quietly (I think I'd been reading too much about Tom and Katie) but the reality was completely different. I mooed a lot and did a fair bit of screaming I think, but I couldn't have done anything differently. Instinct took over completely and I just did what I had to do with each contraction. I felt that it was all taking far too long and I was convinced I must have been pushing for at least two hours (it was actually about 30–40 minutes). All of a sudden, I realised that I was nearly there – the midwife told me to stop pushing otherwise I would tear, but I swear that if I'd been offered a million pounds, I couldn't have stopped. I felt every inch of her come out of my body – the sensation was unlike anything I've ever felt and it seemed to take forever, but finally, she was out.

Time stood still then. The cry that everybody waits for just didn't come. I was still on my hands and knees, biting the headboard of the bed. My legs had cramped up and it was impossible to move and I just assumed that any second now, I would hear a cry and would turn around for the first sight of my precious VBAC baby. Nothing. At some point I was helped on to my back, and by then the paediatricians had been called in. The first time I saw Lydia she was lying completely motionless on the Resuscitaire, with a mask over her face. She was quickly whisked off to intensive care, leaving me lying there, sobbing. I insisted that Peter went with her and was so grateful for the presence of Bushra. I was bleeding very heavily and they were unsure if it was from a tear or if I was haemorrhaging so they asked if I would agree to have syntocinon. Obviously I said yes, but it didn't work so they asked me if I'd agree to it intravenously. I was a little irritated that they were asking me at the time instead of just administering it, but looking back, I had made a big deal in my birth plan about no syntocinon, and about being consulted if they wanted to carry out any interventions, so now I am actually quite impressed that they did as I'd asked. I'm told that the cord had stopped pulsating before it was cut which again I'm pleased about, as Lydia's heart rate was strong from the start. I'm sure that she would have suffered worse damage if it had been cut prematurely.

I had a small tear which they asked if I would have stitched – they had to rule out that as a source of the bleeding, which was still heavy. I was still sucking on the gas and air, fortunately, as being stitched up was deeply unpleasant. Peter recalled returning from SCBU (special care baby unit) to tell me that Lydia was breathing on her own to find me in the stirrups, practically screaming into the gas and air. The registrar explained that she had given me some local anaesthetic to enable her to repair the small tear, to which Peter politely suggested that maybe she hadn't given me quite enough. It took at least four more shots before I stopped feeling the needle.

Lydia was delivered at 2.30am, weighing in at 9lb 10oz, after a very short second stage, with no signs of distress during labour, and no meconium in my waters. We still don't know why she wasn't breathing when she was born, or why she suffered oxygen starvation during my pregnancy/labour/delivery. It was nothing to do with her being a VBAC baby, but just damned bad luck and with hindsight, if I had to do it all over again, I'm sure I would still have opted for VBAC. I feel cheated that it wasn't a happy ever after story, but Lydia was born the way that nature intended and she chose her own birthday. She's beautiful, she has a smile that would melt anyone's heart and I love her. What more can one ask for?

Six months on, she is perfect in every way – we were told to expect signs of cerebral palsy but so far, there is absolutely nothing to suggest that there is anything wrong with her. Another fine example of how wrong doctors can be!

STORY FOUR

A VBAC at home in a birthing pool after two caesareans

Clair had a successful VBAC at home with an independent midwife after two previous caesareans, the first for breech presentation. With her second pregnancy Clair planned a home water birth with NHS midwives but, following a little bleeding after a vaginal examination, the midwife strongly urged her to transfer to hospital and Clair agreed. She told us: *I hope my story offers encouragement to other women. If it wasn't for the ladies on the VBAC group sharing their stories I would never have known that it was possible to have a natural birth after two caesarean sections and I would have missed out on the incredible experience that was the birth of my third child.*

Clair also has ME (Myalgic Encephalomyelitis, also known as Chronic Fatigue Syndrome). She told us: *As far as I know my ME was never an issue. The doctors knew nothing about it and it caused no complications in my pregnancies, but I think I was classed as high risk as no-one knew if it could or would cause any complications.*

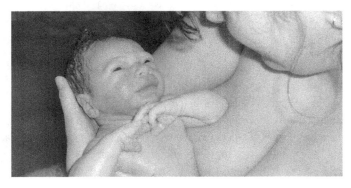

Clair and Samuel, minutes after his birth in the pool

61

Clair's VBAC Story – Samuel

The day after the birth of my second child by caesarean section (CS) the doctor came to see me and said that, as I had had two sections, my next child would be delivered by CS. At my postnatal check up a different doctor asked if I planned to have any more children and, knowing I had planned a home VBAC for my second child, he carefully phrased his words to say it would probably be safer if I were to have another CS. From what I was told I believe the only reason for recommending a third CS was due to me having had two previous sections. There were no complications in either of the surgeries and my two sections were for non-recurring reasons. As far as I know my ME was never an issue. The doctors knew nothing about it and it caused no complications in my pregnancies, but I think I was classed as high risk as no-one knew if it could or would cause any complications.

When I found out I was expecting my third child I was determined to do things differently. After having two previous sections and being told by hospital consultants that my next child would be born by caesarean section, I felt very strongly that I did not want another section and that the NHS could not support me in my wishes so I hired an independent midwife (IM). It was the best decision I ever made. With full support from my IM, I planned a home water birth and I am very happy to say I achieved my goal.

At 6am on 31 January (three days past my due date, 11 days past my hospital due date) I started having regular contractions. I calmly woke my husband and asked him to stay home from work today because I was having the baby. I got up, ate breakfast and then we woke our two children and got them up and dressed. All the while the contractions were getting stronger and closer together so by 7.30am I called my midwife. I called her again at 8.30am and she said she would be on her way over.

We sent my eldest child off to nursery as usual. I stayed very calm, rocking over my birth ball during contractions, watching TV with my youngest child while my husband filled the inflatable birth pool. By 11am the contractions were very strong, the pool was ready and I got in. The contractions faded for a few minutes and my midwife arrived with her student. Then the contractions started again with a vengeance! The water was very helpful, I found it very relaxing between contractions and whilst it didn't make the pains go away it was easier to cope with them than on dry land.

By noon I started getting a strong urge to bear down. It was hard not to push but I tried to breathe through contractions. I started getting tired and asked for gas and air to help me. I had a very strong urge to push and couldn't help myself but there was no sign of baby descending yet. My midwife was incredible throughout, encouraging me and supporting me whilst staying very hands off. She only disturbed me to take my pulse and monitor the baby with the waterproof Sonicaid. She never asked me to change position to do this – she worked around me, and showed me the utmost respect.

Even though I had been pushing for a while things were not progressing so she suggested I get out of the pool and try to empty my bladder. I sat on the toilet for a while but I could not pee so I decided to get back in the pool again. I continued with the gas and air and at around 3pm things started to happen. I got incredible urges to push and the baby started coming down. I felt baby descending and pretty soon his head was visible. I almost pushed his head out but the contraction faded and it slid all the way back in again! I pushed it out with the next contraction. I felt his head between my legs, a very strange sensation! Then the contraction faded and it seemed like forever before the next one came. It did and as I started to push out his body he rotated and kicked me! His little body slithered out and I sat up and picked him up out of the water. I had delivered my son into my own hands. He was pink and alert, his big blue eyes looking at me. He started to breathe right away, he gurgled but didn't cry. It was all very peaceful. My husband and four-and-a-half-year-old son witnessed the birth. My son was very interested and asked if we could keep him. We said yes!

I held our new son in the pool for almost 15 minutes. The placenta wasn't in a hurry to come so we waited until the cord stopped pulsing, tied it with cotton tape and cut it. My husband held our son while I got out of the pool and 90 minutes later delivered the placenta down the toilet. Everyone had tea and biscuits and we settled down with our new family in the comfort of our own home.

Samuel Nathan was born at home in the water at 3.45pm on 31 January 2006. He weighed 8lb 4oz. I was so happy; it was the best experience ever.

I had avoided all hospital pressure for intervention and successfully delivered my son into my own hands. I couldn't believe we had done it! It all seemed so normal and natural, despite it being a home water birth after two sections.

A VBAC at home in a birthing pool after two caesareans

Taryn achieved a successful VBAC at home after a traumatic labour and emergency caesarean with her first child followed by a planned caesarean for her second based on misinformation, despite the fact that she had wanted a vaginal birth.

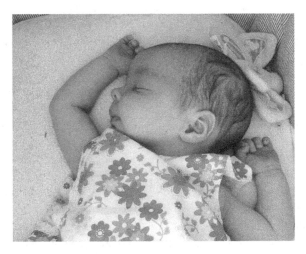

Taryn's VBAC baby Tegan at two weeks old

Taryn's HBA2C story – Tegan

We knew we wanted a third and final baby (final as we know three caesarean sections is meant to be the limit), but I could not face the thought of another caesarean section. When I fell pregnant, and went to my first appointment with my community midwife, she had already put me down for a caesarean section without asking, and was prepared to book a date at that appointment. This time I had access to the Internet from home, and a chance remark from a neighbour asking why I couldn't have it naturally, instead of being told I shouldn't, led me to do some research into the possibility of a home birth.

Then started the gradual process of further research, and sitting down and discussing it with my husband. As soon as I told him of the outcomes of various studies, and the much lower risks than we had been led to believe, and that in fact the size of the baby didn't matter as we had been told in my previous pregnancy, we decided to start preparing to have a home birth. After a lot of discussion we decided that an independent midwife was the way to go, and would try and raise the cash from somewhere. No matter what was said in guidelines, saying we should be supported in whatever our decision for birth was, we knew it would be a struggle to get what we wanted, and would always be on the hospital/midwife's terms rather than a more relaxed approach. I seriously could not face hospital again, and knew that even if by some miracle they let me book a home birth, on the day they would rush me into hospital at the slightest hint of a problem. This was pressure I knew I couldn't take. I knew I needed a more relaxed, less clinical atmosphere if I was going to succeed. If anything was to prove this, at my 20-week appointment the registrar (it was meant to be a consultant!) already assumed I was having a caesarean section. When I said I wanted a VBAC, she said ok, but she didn't recommend it, I would probably fail, and gave me about a 40 per cent success rate, when in reality studies have shown it to be nearer 65–70 per cent. She then booked me in for a growth scan nearer the birth, which we knew I didn't need, and was just a way to get us back in and be pressurised into having a caesarean section. Later, when the independent midwife wrote to the consultant to say she was taking over the care, he sent back quite a sarcastic letter, and cancelled the scan without consulting us. We didn't want the scan anyway, but it really annoyed our midwife, as we should have been consulted first.

We emailed a few midwives, including the Bristol Birth Practice. The first midwife we met was lovely, but we didn't feel completely right with her. Another midwife we chose from the Bristol Birth Practice website was fully booked, but she recommended another. We met them both, and from that minute all the earlier stresses just disappeared. We immediately felt that we had found the right midwife for us, and after they left we were even more determined to find the money.

The pregnancy went well, and the antenatal appointments were a joy. It was amazing having someone come to your house and spend a huge amount of time with you, compared with a community midwife. With all the research we continued doing and all the books our midwife lent us, I was able to work through all the issues of my previous births, and give myself the confidence that my body was not a failure, and that I could give birth naturally. It was an amazing feeling, and my confidence in myself started returning. I had put on a lot of weight, and was very depressed after my first two children. I put on a brave face, just happy that I had my two wonderful boys, but deep inside I felt such a failure. I had already lost the weight to get ready for this pregnancy, and now finally I was starting to feel mentally prepared as well.

We bought our 'Birth Pool in a Box' and enjoyed the rest of the pregnancy, eager for the baby to arrive. For the final few weeks I was having strong Braxton Hicks in the evenings and it became a game of 'will tonight be the night?' Just after my due date, my husband and second son went down with a really bad stomach bug, and we were praying that the birth wouldn't start, as my husband was in no fit state to help, or come in the birth pool with me. I got into bed that night with strong Braxton Hicks, and about an hour later had to get up to go to the toilet. Although I had finished weeing, fluid was still coming out and so I thought might waters might have gone. I fetched a pad, and settled in bed not really believing anything could happen – although I did whisper to my husband that I thought my waters had broken, and we were both really excited, especially as the contractions started to get stronger, and closer, but with no real pattern to them. It was too uncomfortable to sleep, so I got up, baked cakes, and filled the pool between contractions. My husband was also running up to the loo to be ill, and running to my youngest son to help him.

We phoned our family at 4am to come and look after our two sons, and phoned our midwife in the morning. Unfortunately, when she arrived my contractions had died off, so I just relaxed in the pool as I was so tired. As we were unsure as to what was going on, we all decided that it would be a good idea if the midwife gave me an internal. The outcome was that I was still in the very early stages. Our midwife decided it would be best if she left us alone to relax, and came back once labour had started again, which could be anything from hours away to several days.

We tried to sleep during the day, but my contractions kept disturbing me every 20 minutes or so. We went to bed at 9pm, but a horrendously painful contraction woke me at 11pm, and we went back downstairs. From then until about 5am I kept having really painful contractions without any pattern, but which seemed to occur whenever I moved position. I then had an incredible need to get in the birth pool, but my husband who had napped for a couple of hours while my mum looked after me, insisted on phoning the midwife first. Unfortunately he was still a bit drowsy, and didn't realise how things had changed since he went to sleep, and that I had progressed quite a bit. As far as he could tell my contractions were still not regular, but were coming stronger, and more often than before.

I got in the birthing pool, and the contractions accelerated, whilst my husband phoned the midwife back and told her to get over as quickly as possible. It was now just after 8am. Having recovered from his stomach bug, my husband jumped in the pool to help me through the contractions, which had become incredibly painful. Despite several requests from me to take me to hospital, my husband helped me calm down, and we worked through each contraction. My sister was also watching, and I think I scared them both at one point, when I said 'If the midwife doesn't get here I trust you both to help me deliver the baby.' Within no time at all I decided to do my own internal exam, which is something I said I would never want to do, and I felt the head. I told my husband to do the same. It is one of the most incredible things I have ever felt.

At this point my contractions started to change, and my body totally took over. I started to have more time between contractions, my body started to bear down, and I started grunting with each contraction. Shortly after, at 9.30am, our midwife arrived. I started to feel the head coming down, and then moving back up. This is something I had never felt before, and was nothing like I had expected it to be. I was shocked at how well I could feel it, and even asked the midwife if it was normal (I felt so stupid). A second midwife arrived at 10.10am and was quickly briefed on the situation. I then had one huge contraction that I couldn't control, and I felt myself tear, and the head came out. I shouted that this had happened, but I don't think anyone believed it for a couple of seconds, as it happened so quickly. I then said that the head was in my hand, and everyone rushed around to get towels, etc. The rest of the baby was delivered with the next contraction, and the midwife passed her through my legs at 10.16am and onto my chest, where we rubbed her with towels, and made sure her breathing was ok. It was such a relaxed atmosphere, we almost forgot to check to see what sex the baby was. I suggested we had a look, and my husband checked. It was a girl, we couldn't believe it, we even double checked!!! We left the cord pulsing, and she latched on for her first feed. We stayed this way for 20 minutes, whilst we introduced her to our children, and my parents. They then left me to concentrate on delivering the placenta. We decided to get out of the pool, to check how much I had torn, and also investigate where I was bleeding from, as the water was quite dark at this point. Unfortunately as my legs were quite weak, we decided to cut the cord before the placenta arrived, to help me get out of the pool. My husband was extremely happy to finally be able to cut the cord, as he hadn't been able to do it for either of our boys.

Once I had climbed out of the pool, I lay down in some blankets, and fed our daughter while I was checked over. I had two tears, neither of which needed stitches. The placenta was taking a long time to come out, and the midwives were concerned about a pocket of blood behind some tissue so we decided to have the injection to speed up the delivery of the placenta, which was delivered shortly after. The pocket of tissue turned out to be part of the placenta, and not a haematoma.

As a celebratory meal my husband went and got some fresh bread, and a selection of soft cheeses that we had bought ready. It felt like one of the best meals I have ever had in my life. The usual checks were done, and we found out that she was only slightly lighter than either of the boys, at 8lb 11.5oz. At about 12.30 my husband took the baby, whilst the midwife helped me into a nice warm bath. After that we went to bed for the rest of the day. Although I was in pain with the tears, my recovery rate has been amazing compared to either of the caesarean sections, and my energy levels have been a lot higher. When I look back I realise how tired and depressed I was after both my boys. It took me months to recover after them. My daughter has been a much more content baby, and hardly cries – in fact, she has only ever woken for a feed once or twice during the night. More importantly, she came out without any kind of bruising, and has never seemed to be in pain.

We are so glad we went for a home birth, because my waters broke so early that the hospital would never have let me wait so long. That would have meant a third caesarean section. My birth was wonderful and relaxed, and I got to get into my own bed with my husband and baby, without a horrid hospital stay. I also feel as if I could have more children in the future without the fear of a caesarean section hanging over my head. I would never say no to one if it was definitely needed and the baby was in any trouble; but neither would I have one just because the labour was not progressing at the rate a hospital would want. If I have any more children I will be saving for an independent midwife again.

A VBAC at home after four caesareans

Nikki had four caesareans but then achieved a successful VBA4C at home with an independent midwife.

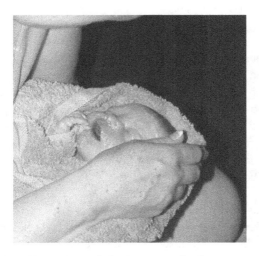

Nikki's VBA4C baby Imogen at birth

Nikki's VBA4C story – Imogen

After a miscarriage at 11 weeks with a fifth baby, we sat down to decide whether or not to try again. We weighed up age, risk of abnormality, cost of starting all over again (monetary as well as emotional) and decided that we would go ahead and let nature take its course – if it was meant to be, then it would happen and be all right; if it wasn't, then it wouldn't.

One month later, I was pregnant. CVS testing showed a healthy (as far as could be ascertained) girl, balancing up the odds in our family.

Now that I knew that the pregnancy appeared to be healthy and fine, I could think about what I wanted from my care and birth. Having had four previous caesareans, I didn't rate my chances too highly within the NHS. Regardless of the way I gave birth I knew that I didn't want to spend the whole pregnancy fighting a system that was not geared up to respecting women's choices and decisions for the pregnancies and births.

So, we made the decision to employ independent midwives and I approached Anna, whom I had spoken to when pregnant before. She was happy to take me on and suggested her mother, Mavis, as second midwife and her colleague Chris, as a third.

At the booking-in visit, we went over everything that had happened with my previous births; but at that time, no explanation could be given as to why the last two babies had decided to go from being very well engaged to oblique presentation during labour. We decided to explore all possibilities and Chris suggested going to see an osteopath in Leeds, to whom she referred all her clients with malpositioned babies. Over subsequent appointments we found that my pelvis and coccyx was fixed on the right-hand side – probably due to a skating accident in my teens. Once this was freed up, the sacroiliac pain I had been putting up with disappeared.

Throughout the pregnancy I felt that I carried this baby much better and easier than with previous ones – maybe due to a more mobile pelvis and the abdominal exercises I had been doing as well. My only concern was that I seemed quite small, even though the baby appeared to be doing well.

So it was full steam ahead and planning for the home birth that I would love to have and hoped to achieve. As I hired out birth pools, I thought it would be rather nice to use one – particularly as it was so close at hand! We put together three birth plans – one for home, one for VBAC in hospital and one for a caesarean birth in hospital. We worked out where to put the birth pool and asked good friends if they would be prepared to step in and look after the children at short notice – I wasn't sure whether or not I would want them there, or even in the house.

As I turned 38 weeks, I started to put things together – a carrier bag of items just in case I needed to put an overnight bag together quickly, doubling up on nappies, breast pads, knickers etc. The baby clothes were brought out and hung up and drawers filled with vests and socks I never thought I would see again. Music was put together and essential oils and carrier oil bought, ready to use. We were going away at the weekend, so the plan was that on our return, the pool would be assembled, the conservatory cleared and everything in place ready for my labour and (hopefully) birth. I was looking forward to the slow build up of labour, to being able to use the pool, to the smell of the oils and the calm, peaceful atmosphere I hoped my baby would be born into. I had been listening to a hypno-birthing CD and wanted to use the music during labour to help give me the encouragement and motivation I needed to believe that this time I could actually give birth.

On the Thursday, I felt rather strange and different and wondered if something was starting. I didn't say anything to Mavis at the antenatal appointment, because I wasn't sure and in any case, if this was early labour, it could stop and start and go on for days. As the pregnancy had been different and this baby was sitting in a different position (on my right hand side, instead of on the left where the others all gravitated to), we had no idea as to how this labour would go. We were guessing that first stage might be quicker – I have laboured with all the previous births – but that second stage might take some time, particularly as I'd never done that bit before.

We were planning to go down to my husband Chris's parents, in Warwickshire, for the weekend and meet up with close friends for dinner. If I was still waiting for things to get going in a week's time, I knew I would regret not going, so off we went on the Saturday.

The two of us spent a rather nice Saturday afternoon mooching about Leamington, buying last-minute items and treating ourselves to a new digital camera. I was getting what I thought were strong Braxton Hicks throughout the day and Chris did ask me if I thought these were the real thing. My reply – 'If I can walk and talk through them then how can it be labour?' I was used to labour starting with period-like contractions, so convinced myself that this was latent labour and could still go on for days and I might as well enjoy myself while I could. Anyway, this just felt niggly and different.

On Saturday evening, we made our way to Rugby to see our friends Kevin and Claire, whom we met during antenatal classes for the last baby (now aged five). I was definitely feeling uncomfortable by now, but passed it off as late-pregnancy niggles – I was determined to enjoy what looked to be a last weekend before the birth. Whilst we sat and chatted, I felt the need to go to the loo and looked as though I was having a show – a lot more mucus than usual, but still I ignored what was going on.

Halfway through dinner I nipped to the loo again as I felt a bit damp – it looked very much as though my waters had started leaking – a very strange situation to be in – it had never happened before. I could no longer ignore what was going on. Claire asked if everything was ok and I asked for a pad, as it looked as though things were happening. I then went to the dining room and asked Chris if he minded missing pudding as I thought we needed to make a move. He later told me that he thought Claire and I had had a falling out! Once he realised that it looked as though this baby was on the way, everything moved quite quickly. We left Kevin and Claire's house with their good luck wishes and made our way back to his parents' house. So we set off and on route I rang Anna to let her know what was happening and that we were making our way from Warwickshire to Yorkshire as quickly as possible. I still felt that this could be latent labour and could go on for hours.

We got back to Chris's parents' house at about 11.15pm. They were very surprised to see us. It was a hot and sticky night, so they had only just got all the children to stay in bed and go to sleep. When we said we were going home because the baby was on the way, they were equally surprised and concerned and wanted us to leave the children behind. The only problem was that our son, Lewis, had an exam on the Monday and it would have been difficult to leave them there and for Chris to try and get back in time to fetch them.

So, we got them all out of bed, put them in the car and left by midnight. All the time, I was feeling more uncomfortable, but still sure that this could go on for hours and I would make it back home with no problems.

At this point, the contractions (which is what they really were) were coming about every 3–5 minutes and lasting about 30 seconds. My only thought was whether I could manage sitting in a car for the next one-and-a-half to two hours whilst we made our way home.

As we made our way up the M1, the contractions started to become stronger and at 12.30pm I rang Anna to let her know that I was having to really concentrate on what was happening with my body. I was also wishing I was at home and not in the front of the car. She reminded me that we could stop off at Mavis's house on the way home if we wanted, to get checked and see what was happening.

I can remember looking at the clock in the car and timing the gap between contractions – about two to three minutes. I was desperate for sleep and found myself dozing in between them. Each contraction needed effort of concentration to focus on them and I found myself not only breathing and trying to relax, but also singing my way up and down a scale as each one increased in intensity. Fortunately it was a clear road and we didn't have any hold-ups, apart from when we thought we were behind a police van, which turned out to be an ambulance.

All the way up, Chris kept asking if I wouldn't just like to go to the nearest hospital – 'No! Just take me home.' I think it would have been grounds for divorce or murder if he had tried to!

At 12.55am, I rang Anna to let her know this was it and we were heading straight for home, we weren't going to Mavis – we'd already passed the junction and were going up the M18. Anna said she would phone Mavis and Chris and then be on her way.

We arrived home at about 1.15am. We had done a two-hour journey in an hour and 15 minutes! By this point I was having massive contractions where my body was doing things I appeared to have no control over – I felt as though I was almost ready to push. All the way through this I kept panicking that the baby had moved and she was in danger and that if she came out vaginally she would be dead. I couldn't believe that this was a straightforward labour and everything was going to plan.

I managed to make it into the front room, having had a massive contraction by the car. I was sure I must have woken the neighbours up (mind you, they might have thought it was someone from the pub round the corner!) I settled in a comfortable position on my knees, draped over the sofa, relieved to have made it home, whilst Chris got the children out of the car. The older two had stayed awake the whole journey – excited, but more so by the speed we were travelling – apparently 100mph at one point. Edward woke up when we got off the motorway and, after being reassured that the noise I was making was because the baby was on her way, became as excited as his brothers. Eloise, on the other hand, was a bit frightened by it and needed some comforting.

Throughout this, I remained convinced that this baby was not in the right position and that I dared not push too soon until I was sure. Chris kept reassuring me that so long as I could feel this hard knobbly bottom, then she hadn't moved.

Anna arrived and got to work. She said she needed to listen to the baby's heartbeat. She found it – just where she was hoping. After feeling round, she told me that the baby was head down and in the right position – moving down well. We managed to get my trousers off. I never realised how difficult it is to move in this late stage of labour. It took a lot of effort to get into a position to take them off and just as I did I remember saying that I thought I had wet myself – no this was the rest of the waters going. Once they were off and I had managed to get back on my knees, Anna asked to do a vaginal examination (the only one I had) and told me that I was fully dilated – she couldn't find any cervix at all. I suspect that I had been like this for some time as I had been having rather pushy contractions that I was fighting – frightened that the baby was not in the right position. I told her I was frightened and scared and that I couldn't do this. Anna told me to put my hand down and feel my baby's head. She put a mirror on the floor so I could see this little dark-haired head appearing and disappearing. She encouraged me – told me that I was going to do this, I was going to have this baby, just as I hoped. I felt then that I could let go and work with these contractions, rather than holding back as I had been doing.

As soon as I did this, I could feel her moving down inside – it was a very strange feeling. I felt determined and focused – in a place I'd hoped to be. All the thoughts of the birth I hoped to have went out of my mind. I didn't care whether there was music, oils and warm fluffy towels. I just wanted to help this baby out. There was a sense of excitement in the room, with Chris rubbing my back and me trying to push with each contraction. I kept trying to keep the towels underneath me and moving them round in a nest of some sorts – it wasn't deliberate, just something I had to do, each time I moved with a contraction. It seemed like a long time, but I had one huge contraction and thought that's it, this baby is coming out NOW!!! I pushed as hard as I could and she shot out. I remember thinking as I was pushing that any minute now Anna is going to tell me to pant as the head comes through, instead of which she was telling me that my baby was born and I could pick her up.

I picked her up in the towels on the floor and gazed at her, completely unbelieving that I had actually just given birth. Anna and Chris were telling me that I had done it, but it just didn't sink in. Chris tried to shoo the children up to bed, but I shouted to him to let them come in and see their new baby sister. It's a fantastic memory – all those faces looking in awe – they didn't see the blood or the mess, they just saw a newborn baby.

So much for the planning – the pool never made it into the house, let alone assembly. The aromatherapy oils were still in our bedroom in their boxes. The nice warm fluffy towels I was going to buy, well they're still in the shop; and the music I was going to put together got no further than the CDs still by the computer, waiting for me to do it. We had to make do with me singing through the contractions! So nothing went the way we hoped and planned, but I still got the home birth and I still gave birth vaginally. Regrets? I should never have gone to Warwickshire!! Then I could have practised what I preach and used different positions and all the stuff I hoped to instead of trying to find a comfortable position in the front seat of the car – not to be recommended in strong labour!

But would I change it? Not a thing. Maybe my labour wouldn't have progressed as fast if I hadn't been away from home. Maybe I wouldn't have coped as well, although I often felt that I wasn't coping at all. Maybe labour would have stalled and I would have needed that transfer to hospital.

But I still can't get used to the fact that I managed to labour and give birth, at home, after four caesareans – something I was told I would never do.

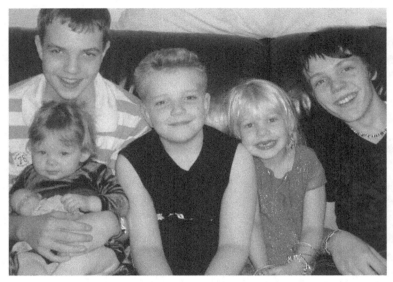

VBAC baby Imogen (18 months) with her caesarean siblings

STORY SEVEN

Two VBACs in hospital after two caesareans

After a caesarean for her first baby, Kate had wanted a VBAC for her second child but was not supported in this by her health care professionals. During her third pregnancy, Kate researched the viability of VBAC and found some supportive health professionals. Despite placental abruption in her first VBAC, Kate went on to have a second successful VBAC completely naturally.

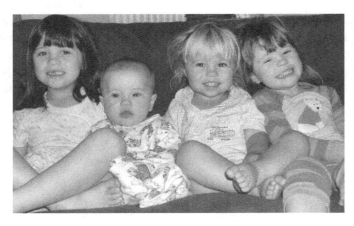

VBAC babies Josephine and Charlie with their caesarean siblings Isabel and Olivia

Kate's 2VBA2C stories – Olivia, Isabel, Charlie and Josephine

On 3 June 2000 we found out that our first IVF (in vitro fertilisation) cycle had failed, and I was devastated. One month later, nature had done her stuff and after a week's denial I did the test that changed my life and saw that blue line! The first thing I did was to enquire about NCT classes: as far as I was concerned it was part of the rite of passage that was pregnancy. My husband and I started the classes after Christmas 2001. I was so excited and, having read every book possible, I knew all the technical terms. We duly went and sat with the other eight expectant parents each Wednesday evening for two hours. Sadly, I was concentrating more on my baby's hiccups than really listening to our teacher and ended up with a section without so much as a twinge, let alone a contraction. I was convinced I would not come home with a live baby and so, when the consultant suggested a caesarean after two failed induction attempts well before my due date (I had a condition called 'polyhydramnios' – too much amniotic fluid), I jumped at the chance. I didn't care how the baby was born, I just wanted a baby! I do not agree with what happened but at the time there was every chance that this would be our only child and I was just desperate to see it. When I hobbled through the front door five days later I felt let down that I hadn't 'given birth'.

When I was pregnant with number two I knew that I wanted to try and give birth naturally and naively thought that the medical profession would help me achieve that. I couldn't have been more wrong. I went into hospital at pretty much the first twinge and was strapped to a monitor. The registrar who attended to me was extremely fierce and, dare I say, aggressive. She certainly wouldn't 'let' me get off the bed and, in my uninformed state, I didn't realise that I could do what I wanted. Isabel was born by caesarean after nine hours of labour having been told I had to be permanently monitored and couldn't move. 'Like a lamb to the slaughter' springs to mind.

My second child was a 'colicky' baby. In hindsight, I am not sure if that is because she picked up on my feelings or that she really wasn't happy in herself, but by the time she was six months old I was on antidepressants, suffering from postnatal depression caused entirely (in my view) by the completely unnecessary section. When she was 11 months old I discovered that I was pregnant for the third time. I had spent pretty much all of Isabel's life researching VBACs so I knew that this time there was no reason that I couldn't do it. I also knew that I HAD to have a vaginal birth. It mattered to me (and still does) that I wasn't going to be cut open again.

Twelve months later I was sitting in my doctor's surgery listening to him saying that both my unborn baby and I would die if I attempted a VBA2C. He was wrong! I surfed the Internet daily for any information and statistics that would further my cause. I was determined to birth my own baby. We arranged to attend an NCT day course. I actually paid some attention and came out of there empowered. I knew that my body could do it, I just had to find some health professionals who would support me. We decided at 30 weeks to try a different hospital, where we met my consultant who agreed with us, encouraging me to have a water birth if I wanted. Charlie was born after a labour lasting one hour, culminating in a placental abruption and an episiotomy. I walked out of hospital with my husband 12 hours after Charlie was born – an impossibility after a section.

Ten months later I was pregnant with our fourth baby. I was keen on a home birth this time, especially as Charlie had arrived so quickly. Again we were referred to the hospital where I had my VBAC, mainly to see the consultant and discuss the possibility of another abruption. I was slightly more at risk but not dangerously so – I had a 0.1 per cent chance of uterine rupture and a 4 per cent chance of abruption. Our plans were full steam ahead for the HBA2C. Again we booked in for a two-day NCT course. I wanted to cover all options so that if I ended up with another section, it wasn't because I wasn't prepared for the birth. Towards the end of the pregnancy the baby couldn't make up its mind which way round it wanted to be, going from head down to breech to transverse. My consultant said that even I couldn't give birth to a sideways baby, although he was happy to support me birthing a breech one. We got a bit nervous so it was agreed that I would go and stay in hospital around the time we thought the baby would arrive. Charlie (my previous VBAC baby) was 11 days late, so I felt (and the consultant agreed) that this one wouldn't make an appearance any earlier, although I lived in hope. I ended up being admitted 14 days overdue when things looked as though they might kick off at any moment.

Three days later I was still in hospital having had a very lazy weekend. I began to have a few twinges around lunchtime on the Monday. By the early evening the twinges had become regular and it was obvious that something was going to happen that evening. My husband Philip arrived at 6.45pm and apart from a midwife trying to tell him he wasn't allowed on the ward (I told him and her that he was) things were going ok. I was using the TENS machine by now, which was great and enabled me to carry on watching the Commonwealth Games without too much bother. After about half an hour, I decided that I wanted to go over to the labour ward as the gas and air was beginning to sound appealing. However, when I went to the loo I realised that the baby was on its way. I panicked slightly and, screaming for Philip, I pulled the emergency cord (always wanted to do that). Philip and a midwife burst in (fortunately I had forgotten to lock the door) and bundled me into a wheelchair with a cot sheet covering my modesty!

So our fourth child and third daughter was born after an official labour of one hour with a further five minutes of pushing. She was our only completely natural birth and was the largest (a whopping 10lb 12oz or 4.86kg). I gave birth half kneeling, half squatting. She was born at 8.15pm, and at five to midnight the three of us left the hospital. What an amazing way to complete our family – four is plenty for us.

Charlie (number three) was very much my 'cure' and I am very proud of my achievement of both VBA2Cs which my husband and I fought so hard to get. It saddens me that, even now, people are amazed to hear that I was 'allowed' to have a natural delivery and also that I have had to spend some of my last two pregnancies fighting to get the birth that I was cheated out of with Isabel and to a smaller extent Olivia (number one).

I am horrified when so-called celebrities say how much easier a section is compared to natural birth. I do understand that sometimes there is a genuine need for a section but in my view it is not the easy option. If I had my time again I would never have agreed so readily to that first one.

We hope that these birth stories give you hope and encouragement to see that VBAC is a safe and viable option for you in most cases. On pages 94–5 you will find a list of useful contacts – organisations and websites where you can find more information and the practical support you may need. Good luck!

References

1 National Institutes of Health, *Cesarean Childbirth*, US Department of Health and Human Services, Public Health Service, publication No. 82-2067, Washington DC: US Government Printing Office, 1982.

2 DHHS Department of Health and Human Services, *Healthy People 2000*, Washington DC: DHSS Publications No. (PHS) 91-50212, 1991.

3 Francome, C. and Savage, W. 'Caesarean Section in Britain and the United States 12% or 24%: is either too high?' *Social Science and Medicine* 1993, 37(10):1199–1218.

4 Royal College of Obstetricians and Gynaecologists, *Birth After Previous Caesarean Birth*, Green-top Guideline No.45, February 2007, London: RCOG, paragraph 6.2.

5 Thomas, J. and Paranjothy, S. *National Sentinel Caesarean Section Audit Report*, Royal College of Obstetricians and Gynaecologists Clinical Effectiveness Support Unit, London: RCOG Press, 2001.

6 Singh, T., Justin, C.W. and Haloob, R.K. 'An audit on trends of vaginal delivery after one previous caesarean section', *Journal of Obstetrics and Gynaecology* 2004, 24(2):135–8.

7 Re MB (an adult: medical treatment) [1997] 2 FCR 541, CA.

8 Churchill, H., Savage, W. and Francome, C. *Caesarean Birth in Britain, Revised and Updated*. London: Middlesex University Press, 2006.

9 WHO World Health Organisation, 'Appropriate Technology for Birth', *The Lancet* 1985, 331:436–7.

10 Thomas, J. and Paranjothy, S. *National Sentinel Caesarean Section Audit Report*, Royal College of Obstetricians and Gynaecologists Clinical Effectiveness Support Unit, London: RCOG Press, 2001.

11 Placek, P.J. and Taffel, S.M. 'Vaginal birth after cesarean (VBAC) in the 1980s', *American Journal of Public Health* 1988, 78(5):512–5.

12 Enkin, M., Keirse, M.J.N.C., Neilson, J., et al. *A Guide to Effective Care in Pregnancy and Childbirth, third edition*, Oxford: Oxford University Press, 2000.

13 Grinstead, J. and Grobman, W.A. 'Induction of labor after one prior cesarean: predictors of vaginal delivery', *Obstetrics & Gynecology* 2004, 103(3): 534–8.

14 Odibo, A.O. and Macones, G.A. 'Current concepts regarding vaginal birth after caesarean delivery', *Current Opinion in Obstetrics and Gynecology* 2003, 15(6):479–82.

15 Landon, M.B., Leindecker, S., Spong, C.Y., et al. 'The MFMU Cesarean Registry: Factors affecting the success of trial of labor after previous cesarean delivery', *American Journal of Obstetrics and Gynecology* 2005, 193:1016–23.

16 Brill, Y. and Windrim, R. 'Vaginal birth after caesarean section: review of antenatal predictors of success', *Journal of Obstetrics and Gynaecology of Canada* 2003, 25(4):275–86.

17 Enkin, M., Keirse, M.J.N.C., Neilson, J., et al. *A Guide to Effective Care in Pregnancy and Childbirth, third edition*, Oxford: Oxford University Press, 2000.

18 Grinstead, J. and Grobman, W.A. 'Induction of labor after one prior cesarean: predictors of vaginal delivery', *Obstetrics & Gynecology* 2004, 103(3) 534–8.

19 Author not given, 'Electronic Foetal Heart Rate Monitoring: Research Guidelines for Interpretation', *American Journal of Obstetrics and Gynecology* 1997, 177(6):1385–90.

20 Blanchette, H., et al. 'Is Vaginal Birth After Cesarean Safe? Experience at a community hospital', *American Journal of Obstetrics and Gynecology* 2001, 184:1478–87.

21 Landon, M.B., Leindecker, S., Spong, C.Y., et al. 'The MFMU Cesarean Registry: Factors affecting the success of trial of labor after previous cesarean delivery', *American Journal of Obstetrics and Gynecology* 2005, 193:1016–23.

22 Macones, G.A., Peipert, J., Nelson, D.B., et al. 'Maternal complications with vaginal birth after cesarean delivery: A Multicenter study', *American Journal of Obstetrics and Gynecology* 2005, 193:1656–62.

23 Gyamfi, C., Juhasz, G., Gyamfi, P., et al. 'Increased success of trial of labor after previous vaginal birth after caesarean', *Obstetrics and Gynecology* 2004, 104(4):715–19.

24 ACNM American College of Nurse Midwives, 'Vaginal birth after previous caesarean section', *Clinical Bulletin* 2004, 49(1):68–74.

25 Johnson, P.G. and Wiencek, V. 'The relationship between amniotomy, provider type and caesarean section in a university medical centre', *Canadian Journal of Midwifery Research and Practice* 2005, 4(2):25–9.

26 Walton, C., Yiannousiz, K. and Gatsby, H. 'Promoting midwifery-led care within an obstetric-led unit', *British Journal of Midwifery* 2005, 13(12):750–54.

27 NICE National Institute for Clinical Excellence, *Caesarean Section, National Collaborating Centre for Women's and Children's Health*, Clinical Guideline, London: RCOG Press, 2004.

28 Personal communication from British obstetrician, 2007.

29 Enkin, M., Keirse, M.J.N.C., Neilson, J., et al. *A Guide to Effective Care in Pregnancy and Childbirth, third edition*, Oxford: Oxford University Press, 2000.

30 Cheung, V.Y.T. 'Sonographic measurement of the lower uterine segment thickness in women with previous caesarean section', *Journal of Obstetrics and Gynecology of Canada* 2005, 27(7):674–81.

31 Enkin, M., Keirse, M.J.N.C., Neilson, J., et al. *A Guide to Effective Care in Pregnancy and Childbirth, third edition*, Oxford: Oxford University Press, 2000.

32 Macones, G.A., Peipert, J., Nelson, D.B., et al. 'Maternal complications with vaginal birth after cesarean delivery: A Multicenter study', *American Journal of Obstetrics and Gynecology* 2005, 193:1656–62.

33 Enkin, M., Keirse, M.J.N.C., Neilson, J., et al. *A Guide to Effective Care in Pregnancy and Childbirth, third edition*, Oxford: Oxford University Press, 2000.

34 Ibid.

35 Phipps, M., Watabe, B., Clemons, J.L., et al. 'Risk factors for bladder injury during caesarean delivery', *Obstetrics and Gynecology* 2005, 105(1):156–60.

36 Macones, G.A., Peipert, J., Nelson, D.B., et al. 'Maternal complications with

vaginal birth after cesarean delivery: A Multicenter study', *American Journal of Obstetrics and Gynecology* 2005, 193:1656–62.

37   Ibid.

38   Gould, D., et al. 'Emergency Obstetric Hysterectomy – an increasing incidence', *Journal of Obstetrics and Gynaecology* 1999, 19:580–3.

39   Fogelson, N.S., Menard, M.K., Hulsey, T., et al. 'Neonatal impact of elective repeat cesarean delivery at term: A comment on patient choice cesarean delivery', *American Journal of Obstetrics and Gynecology* 2005, 192:1433–6.

40   MacDorman, M.F., Declercq, E., Menacker, F., et al. 'Infant and Neonatal Mortality for Primary Cesarean and Vaginal Births to Women with "No Indicated Risk", United States, 1998–2001 Birth Cohorts', *Birth* 2006, 33(3):175–82.

41   Villar, J., Valladares, E.I., Wojdyla, D., et al. 'WHO 2005 global survey on maternal and perinatal health research group, Caesarean delivery rates and pregnancy outcomes: the 2005 WHO global survey on maternal and perinatal health in Latin America', *Lancet* 2006, 367:1819–29.

42   Wen, S.W., Rusen, I.D., Walker, M., et al. 'Comparison of maternal mortality and morbidity between trial of labor and elective cesarean section among women with previous cesarean delivery', *American Journal of Obstetrics and Gynecology* 2004, 191:1263–9.

43   DoH Department of Health, *Why mothers die 2000–2002. Report on confidential enquiries into maternal mortality in the United Kingdom*, London: RCOG Press, 2004, table 1.11.

44   Getahun, D., Oyeoese, Y., Salihu et al. 'Previous cesarean delivery and risk of placenta previa and placental abruption', *Obstetrics and Gynecology* 2006, 107(4):771–8.

45   Gaskin, I.M. 'A new VBAC concern', *Birth Gazette* 2000, 16(2):42.

46   Getahun, D., Oyeoese, Y., Salihu et al. 'Previous cesarean delivery and risk of placenta previa and placental abruption', *Obstetrics and Gynecology* 2006, 107(4):771–8.

47   Homebirth.org, *The VBAC Pages, Vaginal Birth After Caesarean?* 2001 http://www.homebirth.org/vbac.htm [Accessed 21 April 2005].

48   Landon, M.B., Leindecker, S., Spong, C.Y., et al. 'The MFMU Cesarean Registry: factors affecting the success of trial of labor after previous cesarean delivery', *American Journal of Obstetrics and Gynecology* 2005, 193:1016–23.

49   Enkin, M., Keirse, M.J.N.C., Neilson, J., et al. *A Guide to Effective Care in Pregnancy and Childbirth, third edition*, Oxford: Oxford University Press, 2000.

50   Bujold, E., Gauthier, R.J. 'Should we allow a trial of labor after a previous cesarean for dystocia in the second stage of labor?' *Obstetrics and Gynecology* 2001, 98(4):652–5.

51   Brill, Y. and Windrim, R. 'Vaginal birth after caesarean section: review of antenatal predictors of success', *Journal of Obstetrics and Gynaecology of Canada* 2003, 25(4):275–86.

52   Ibid.

53   Cahill, A., Stamilio, D.M., Pare, E., et al. 'Vaginal birth after cesarean (VBAC)

attempt in twin pregnancies: Is it safe?' *American Journal of Obstetrics and Gynecology* 2005, 193:1050–5.

54 Varner, M.W., Leindecker, S., Spong, C.Y., et al. 'The maternal-fetal medicine unit cesarean registry: Trial of labor with a twin gestation', *American Journal of Obstetrics and Gynecology*, 2005, 193:135–40.

55 Haest, K.M.J., Roumen, F.J.M.E. and Nijhuis, J.G. 'Neonatal and maternal outcomes in twin gestations ≥32 weeks according to the planned mode of delivery', *European Journal of Obstetrics and Gynecology and Reproductive Biology* 2005, 123(1):17–21.

56 Ginsberg, N.A. and Levine, E.M. 'Delivery of the second twin', *International Journal of Gynecology and Obstetrics* 2005, 91:217–20.

57 Sindu, K., Srinivas, S.K., Stamilio, et al. 'Safety and success of vaginal birth after cesarean delivery in patients with preeclampsia', *American Journal of Perinatology* 2006, 23:145–52.

58 Bujold, E., Hammoud, A.O., Hendler, I., et al. 'Trial of labor in patients with previous cesarean section: does maternal age influence the outcome?' *American Journal of Obstetrics and Gynecology* 2004, 190(4):1113–18.

59 Carroll, C.S. Sr., Magann, E.F., Chauhan, S.P., et al. 'Vaginal Birth after Cesarean Section versus repeat cesarean delivery: weight-based outcomes', *American Journal of Obstetrics & Gynecology* 2003, 188:1516–20.

60 Durnwald, C.P., Ehrenberg, H.M., Mercer, B.M. 'The impact of maternal obesity and weight gain on vaginal birth after cesarean section success', *American Journal of Obstetrics and Gynecology* 2004, 191(3):954–7.

61 Brill, Y. and Windrim, R. 'Vaginal birth after caesarean section: review of antenatal predictors of success', *Journal of Obstetrics and Gynaecology of Canada* 2003, 25(4):275–86.

62 Goodall, P.T., Ahn, J.T., Chapa, J.B., et al. 'Obesity as a risk factor for failed trial of labor in patients with previous caesarean delivery', *American Journal of Obstetrics and Gynecology*, 192(5) May 2005: 1423–6.

63 Odibo, A.O. and Macones, G.A. 'Current concepts regarding vaginal birth after caesarean delivery', *Current Opinion in Obstetrics and Gynecology* 2003, 15(6):479–82.

64 Landon, M.B., Leindecker, S., Spong, C.Y., et al. 'The MFMU Cesarean Registry: Factors affecting the success of trial of labor after previous cesarean delivery', *American Journal of Obstetrics and Gynecology* 2005, 193:1016–23.

65 Kayani, S.A. and Alfirevic, Z. 'Uterine rupture after induction of labour in women with previous caesarean section', *British Journal of Obstetrics and Gynaecology* 2004, 112:451–5.

66 McDonough, M.S., Osterweil, P. and Guise, J.M. 'The benefits and risk of inducing labour in patients with prior caesarean delivery: a systematic review', *British Journal of Obstetrics and Gynaecology* 2005, 112:1007–15.

67 Ibid.

68 Aslan, H., et al. 'Uterine rupture associated with misoprostol labor induction in women with previous caesarean delivery', *European Journal of Obstetrics and Gynecology and Reproductive Biology* 2004, 113(1):45–8.

69 Ardiet, E., Subtil, D. and Puech, F. 'Cervical ripening with dinoprostone gel and previous cesarean delivery', *International Journal of Gynecology and Obstetrics* 2005, 91:260–61.

70 Bujold, E., Blackwell, S.C., Hendler, I., et al. 'Modified Bishop's score and induction of labor in patients with a previous cesarean delivery', *American Journal of Obstetrics and Gynecology* 2004, 191:1644–48.

71 Pathedey, S.D., Van Woerden, H.C. and Jenkinson, S.D. 'Induction of labour after a previous caesarean section: a retrospective study in a district general hospital', *Journal of Obstetrics and Gynaecology* 2005, 25(7):662–65.

72 Brill, Y. and Windrim, R. 'Vaginal birth after caesarean section: review of antenatal predictors of success', *Journal of Obstetrics and Gynaecology of Canada* 2003, 25(4):275–86.

73 Elkousy, M.A., Sammel, M., Stevens, E., et al. 'The effect of birthweight on vaginal birth after cesarean delivery success rates', *American Journal of Obstetrics and Gynecology* 2003, 188(3):824–30.

74 Brill, Y. and Windrim, R. 'Vaginal birth after caesarean section: review of antenatal predictors of success', *Journal of Obstetrics and Gynaecology of Canada* 2003, 25(4):275–86.

75 Coassolo, K.M., Stamilio, D.M. and Pare, E. 'Safety and efficacy of vaginal birth after caesarean attempts at or beyond 40 weeks of gestation', *Obstetrics and Gynaecology* 2005, 106(4):700–6.

76 Marchiano, D., et al. 'Diet controlled gestational diabetes mellitus does not influence the success rates for vaginal delivery after caesarean delivery', *American Journal of Obstetrics & Gynecology* 2004, 190(3): 790–6.

77 Sharma, S. and Thorpe-Beeston, J.G. 'Trial of vaginal delivery following three previous caesarean sections', *British Journal of Obstetrics and Gynaecology* 2002, 109(3):350–1.

78 Macones, G.A., Cahill, A., Pare, E., et al. 'Obstetric outcomes in women with two prior cesarean deliveries: is vaginal birth after cesarean a viable option?' *American Journal of Obstetrics and Gynecology* 2005, 192(4):1223–9.

79 Churchill, H., Savage, W. and Francome, C. *Caesarean Birth in Britain, Revised and Updated.* London: Middlesex University Press, 2006.

80 NICE National Institute for Clinical Excellence, *Caesarean Section, National Collaborating Centre for Women's and Children's Health, Clinical Guideline,* London: RCOG Press, 2004.

81 Churchill, H. *Caesarean Birth: Experience, Practice and History,* Manchester: Books for Midwives Press,1999.

82 Bucklin, B.A. 'Vaginal birth after cesarean delivery', *Anesthesiology* 2003, 99(6):1444–8.

83 Dodd, J. and Crowther, C.A. 'Vaginal birth after caesarean section: a survey of practice in Australia and New Zealand', *Australian and New Zealand Journal of Obstetrics and Gynaecology* 2003, 43(3):226–31.

84 Dauphinee, J.D. 'VBAC: safety for the patient and nurse', *Journal of Obstetric, Gynecological and Neonatal Nursing* 2004, 33(1):105–15.

85 Leiberman, E., Ernst, E., Rooks, J., et al. 'Results of the national study of vaginal birth after caesarean in birth centers', *Obstetrics and Gynecology* 2004, 104(5):933–42.

86 Latendresse, G., Aikins Murphy, P. and Fullerton, J.T. 'A description of the management and outcomes of vaginal birth after cesarean birth in the homebirth setting', *Journal of Midwifery and Women's Health* 2005, 50(5):386–91.

87 Chamberlain, G., Wraight, A. and Crowley, P. (eds) 'National Birthday Trust – Report of the Confidential Enquiry into Home Births', *Practising Midwife* 1999, 2(7):35–9.

88 Thewlis, S. 'Midwives and Home Birth', *Nursing and Midwives Circular* 8–2006, p.4. http://www.nmc-uk.org/aFrameDisplay.aspx?DocumentID=1680 [Accessed 08 April 2007].

89 Cleary-Goldman, J., Cornelisse, K., Simpson, L.L., et al. 'Previous cesarean delivery: understanding and satisfaction with mode of delivery in a subsequent pregnancy in patients participating in a formal vaginal birth after cesarean counselling program', *American Journal of Perinatology* 2005, 22(4):217–21.

90 Dunn, E.A. and O'Herlihy, C. 'Comparison of maternal satisfaction following vaginal delivery after caesarean section and caesarean section after previous vaginal delivery', *European Journal of Obstetrics and Gynaecology and Reproductive Biology* 2005, 121:56–60.

91 McGarry, J.A. 'The management of patients previously delivered by caesarean section', *Journal of Obstetrics and Gynaecology of the British Commonwealth* 1969, 76:137–43.

Abbreviations

ACOG American College of Obstetricians and Gynecologists
ARM Artificial rupture of the membranes
BMI Body mass index
CPD Cephalopelvic disproportion
CSR Caesarean section rate
CVS Chorionic villus sampling
FD Fetal distress
FTP Failure to progress
G & A Gas and air
GH Gestational hypertension
HBAC Vaginal birth at home after previous caesarean (HBA2C is a home vaginal birth after two caesareans)

IM Independent midwife
IVF In vitro fertilisation
NICE National Institute for Clinical Excellence (UK)
NICHD National Institute of Child Health and Human Development (USA)
ME Myalgic encephalomyelitis, also known as chronic fatigue syndrome
NHS National Health Service
PET Pre-eclampsia
RCOG Royal College of Obstetricians and Gynaecologists (UK)
TENS Transcutaneous electrical nerve stimulation
US / USA United States of America
VBAC Vaginal birth after caesarean
VBA2C Vaginal birth after two caesareans
VE Vaginal examination

Glossary

Anaemia – A condition in which the blood is deficient in red blood cells.

Anterior lip (of cervix) – When part of the cervix remains in front of the baby's head during delivery.

Body mass index (BMI) – A calculation using a person's weight and height to determine the amount of fat they carry.

Braxton Hicks – Rhythmic uterine muscle activity which occurs during the course of a pregnancy which usually cause no pain.

Chorionic villus sampling (CVS) – A prenatal test that detects chromosomal abnormalities such as Down's syndrome.

Clavicle – Collar bone.

Coccyx – The last bone at the base of the spine.

Doula – A woman experienced in childbirth (not necessarily medically qualified) who provides advice, information and emotional support to a mother before, during and just after childbirth.

Effacing – Shortening, softening and thinning of the cervix during labour.

Episiotomy – A cut made into the perineum, using surgical scissors, to enlarge the vaginal opening before delivery. It can be performed by either a midwife or a doctor.

Fetal distress – When the baby in the uterus is short of oxygen. It can be diagnosed by changes in the baby's heart rate and sometimes from the baby passing meconium into the amniotic fluid, as well as by fetal blood sampling.

Fetus – The baby before it is born. In human development, the period after the seventh or eighth week of pregnancy is the fetal period. (Sometimes spelt 'foetus'.)

Haematoma – A localised collection of blood, usually clotted, in an organ, space or tissue, due to a break in the wall of a blood vessel.

Lay – as in 'lay women', means 'not professional'; that is, the general public.

Mal-positioned – When referring to babies in the womb meaning not in the usual vertex (head-down) position for birth.

Meconium – The waste products of development retained in the baby's intestines before birth. If the baby passes meconium during labour, the amniotic fluid turns brown and this can be, but is not always, a sign of fetal distress.

Misoprostol – A synthetic prostaglandin licensed and used to treat stomach ulcers and in the induction of medical abortion. It has been used despite being unlicensed to induce labour. The manufacturers warned against this in 2000, especially in women with a uterine scar.

Oblique (presentation) – When the baby is lying with its head or bottom under the mother's ribs on the left or right and its other end near the bone above the hip.

Pfannenstiel's cut – A long horizontal abdominal incision made below the line of the pubic hair (also known as the bikini-line cut).

Pre-eclampsia – A condition arising during pregnancy. Symptoms are increased blood pressure often accompanied by swelling of the limbs and protein in the urine. The only 'cure' is delivery of the baby, by early induction of labour or by caesarean if the condition is severe and the cervix unfavourable. If left untreated, it can cause fits in the mother and cut off the oxygen supply to her baby.

Premature – Born after a gestation period of less than 37 weeks.

Prostaglandins – Naturally occurring substances, which are made by the body and short-lived. Many are involved in menstruation. Synthetic substances similar to, but not exactly the same, are used to induce labour.

Pulmonary vein – Vein carrying oxygenated blood from the lungs.

Randomised controlled trial – A clinical trial in which the subjects are randomly distributed into groups which are either subjected to the experimental procedure (such as use of a drug or procedure/treatment) or which serve as controls, i.e. no treatment.

Resuscitaire – A raised angled platform with good lighting, a heater, suction and oxygen tubes, on which the baby is placed so midwives and doctors can help if the baby does not breathe immediately.

Rupture – The forcible tearing apart of tissue.

Sacroiliac – Relating to or affecting the joint between the sacrum and the ileum, one of the bones in the pelvic girdle.

Syntocinon – A drug containing a synthetic version of the naturally occurring hormone oxytocin. Synthetic oxytocin is used to induce labour for medical reasons, or if labour has not started naturally following spontaneous rupture of the membranes (breaking of the waters). After the baby has been born, Syntocinon may be given to stimulate contractions that help push out the placenta and prevent heavy bleeding.

TENS (Transcutaneous Electrical Nerve Stimulation) – A low-tech form of pain relief which a woman can use on herself by means of a small, hand-held, battery-operated machine. TENS works by means of two pairs of electrodes taped to the woman's lower back, transmitting a signal which works in two ways to reduce the level of pain from contractions. The first is by interfering with the signals being transmitted to the brain; the second by promoting the production of the body's naturally occurring pain-killers, endorphins.

Thromboembolism – The condition where blood clots in a vein which may be superficial or a deep vein thrombosis in the leg. If the clots break loose they can be carried by the blood stream from the site of origin to plug another vessel. If this is the pulmonary vein it is very dangerous.

Ventouse – A method of helping a mother to deliver her baby, used by doctors or specially trained midwives. A cup is attached by a strong tube to an electric pump. The cup is put on the baby's head and a vacuum created by the pump to keep it in place. With one hand on the baby's head, the doctor pulls on the tube during a contraction to deliver the baby. If not much pulling is needed, a soft silicone cup can be used which causes less bruising to the baby's head. The mother may need a small episiotomy or none at all, depending on the position of the baby.

Further information for parents

Balaskas, J. *Active Birth: The new approach to giving birth naturally*, revised edition, Harvard Common Press, 1992.
How to prepare for an active birth.

Enkin, M., Keirse, M., Neilson, J., Crowther, C., Dudley, L., Hodnett, E. and Hofmeyr, J. *A Guide to Effective Care in Pregnancy and Childbirth*, third edition, Oxford University Press, 2000.
A summary of research findings on all aspects of maternity care.

MIDIRS (Midwives Information and Resource Service) Leaflets for patients and professionals: *Caesarean Birth and VBAC*, Informed Choice Series, Leaflet No 17.
A short leaflet containing information on caesarean birth in general and a section on VBAC available through MIDIRS. Address: MIDIRS, Freepost, 9 Elmdale Road, Clifton, Bristol, BS8 1ZZ. Website: www.infochoice.org

NCT Information Sheet: *Vaginal birth after caesarean*.
A short information sheet on VBAC, accessed through the NCT (see below).

Organisations

Association for Improvements in the Maternity Services (AIMS)
Helpline: 0870 765 1433
Website: www.aims.org.uk
Voluntary pressure group offering support with regard to parents' rights, complaints procedures and choices for maternity care.

National Childbirth Trust
Alexandra House, Oldham Terrace, Acton, London W3 6NH
Tel: 0870 770 3236
Website: www.nct.org.uk
Email: enquiries@nct.org.uk

Over 320 local branches throughout the United Kingdom with networks of informal support, including antenatal teachers, breastfeeding counsellors and postnatal support groups. Local branches will have information about what sort of service to expect from local maternity services and will have details of local support groups for home birth and for women who have had or are expecting to have a caesarean. ParentAbility provides information for parents with disabilities or medical conditions and puts them in touch with each other.

VBAC Information and Support, c/o Caroline Spear, 50 Whiteways, North Bersted, Bognor Regis, West Sussex, PO22 9AS
Tel: 01243 868440

Network of volunteers offering information and support for women wanting a vaginal birth after a previous caesarean.

Websites

www.birthchoiceuk.com

>   Explains options and gives information to help you make choices about where to have your baby and who should look after you in labour.

www.childbirth.org

>   Promotes birth as a natural process. Provides links to other useful sites.

www.homebirth.org.uk

>   Information about home birth for parents and professionals, including a page on VBAC.

www.nct.org.uk

>   NCT offers support in pregnancy, childbirth and early parenthood. They aim to give every parent the chance to make informed choices.

www.vbac.org.uk

>   These pages were initially written after requests from women considering home VBAC, but they are also relevant for those planning hospital births.

Index

Printed in the USA
CPSIA information can be obtained
at www.ICGtesting.com
LVHW011130090824
787694LV00003B/371

9 781905 177240